Headache
SIMPLIFIED

D1276792

Dawn A. Marcus, MD

tfm Publishing Limited, Castle Hill Barns, Harley, Nr Shrewsbury, SY5 6LX, UK. Tel: +44 (0)1952 510061; Fax: +44 (0)1952 510192 E-mail: nikki@tfmpublishing.com; Web site: www.tfmpublishing.com

Design & Typesetting: Nikki Bramhill BSc Hons Dip Law
First Edition: September © 2008

ISBN: 978 1 903378 67 0

Printed by Gutenberg Press Ltd., Gudja Road, Tarxien, PLA 19, Malta. Tel: +356 21897037; Fax: +356 21800069.

Contents

Preface

Dramatic changes have evolved in the field of headache over the last several years as researchers have identified clear neural changes that result in the complex symptomatology experienced in common headache disorders. Better understanding of physiological changes producing the symptom of headache and common syndromes like migraine has resulted in improved credibility of this commonly reported and often disabling complaint. Improved validity for headache has not only improved acceptance of this symptom as legitimate by patients and healthcare providers, but has resulted in a wealth of new research into more effective methods for evaluating and treating headache.

Increased information available to patients through direct-to-consumer marketing and internet resources has improved patient awareness that headache should not simply be endured, but should be managed as other accepted health conditions. Unfortunately, headache often accompanies a complex assortment of ailments, requiring careful evaluation to establish an accurate diagnosis and effective treatment plan. Headache patients can present a unique set of challenges as this pain symptom may affect many areas of their lives, including daily lifestyle patterns, work ability, and plans for pregnancy. This book is designed to provide the busy clinician with a comprehensive understanding of headache pathophysiology and diagnosis, along with practical tools to distinguish common and uncommon headache syndromes and provide effective treatment. Up-to-date information is provided to recognize important characteristics of headache epidemiology and impact, along with techniques for reducing headache occurrence and disability. The reader will be taken through the steps for differentiating primary from secondary headache disorders, and offered hints for identifying uncommon or rare headache conditions. The role of important comorbid conditions, such as cardiovascular disease, epilepsy, fibromyalgia, and mood disorder are also detailed.

This book provides practical, evidence-based treatment recommendations that encompass traditional medical treatments, as well as complementary and alternative therapies. State-of-the-art, emerging therapies for both acute treatment and prevention of headaches are also detailed. Utilizing the information provided in this book will allow the clinician to knowledgably offer patients a full complement of therapeutic recommendations for both common and uncommon headache conditions. Special sections describing headaches in children and adolescents, women during pregnancy, and adults during geriatric years complete this comprehensive reference. Heavy reliance on algorithms, figures, tables, and the latest research provide an up-to-date resource that is easy to access in the clinic.

Dawn A. Marcus, MD
Professor, Department of Anesthesiology,
Pain Evaluation and Treatment Institute,
University of Pittsburgh, Pittsburgh, USA

Glossary of terms

Chapter 1

Term	Definition
Epidemiology terms	
Incidence	Onset of new cases of a condition. How many new cases develop within a population during a specified time.
Prevalence	Proportion of a population with a condition. How many people currently have a condition.
Acute	New onset condition or symptom.
Chronic	Condition or symptom that has been present for ≥3 months.
Headache categories	
Primary headache	Head pain is the primary symptom of the disorder and not a symptom of another medical illness.
Secondary headache	Head pain occurs as a symptom of another condition or illness.
Headache diagnoses	
Migraine	Intermittent, disabling headache associated with sensitivity to lights and noises or nausea.
Tension-type headache	Intermittent or constant, non-disabling headache.
Cluster headache	Excruciating, recurring brief episodes of unilateral peri-orbital pain.

Post-trauma headache	Headache occurring after head injury with concussion.
Medication overuse headache	Headache aggravated by daily or near daily analgesic or other medication use. Previously called *rebound* headache.

Chapter 2

Term	**Definition**
Historical terms	
Phonophobia	Extreme sensitivity to *normal conversational speech*. Patients usually need to turn off radio and television and seek quiet.
Photophobia	Extreme sensitivity to *normal room lighting*. Patients usually close blinds and turn off lights. They may cover eyes with a washcloth.
Physical examination terms	
Papilledema	Swelling of the optic head seen on fundoscopic examination with the ophthalmoscope. Generally signifies increased intracranial pressure.
Range of motion (ROM)	Active ROM describes how far a patient can move his or her neck, extremities, or joints. Passive ROM describes joint restrictions identified when the examiner moves joints in a relaxed patient. Abnormalities with passive ROM suggest joint disturbance, while restrictions with active ROM may result from pain restrictions, muscle spasm, or joint dysfunction.

Specialized testing terms

CT

Computed tomography creates computer-generated brain images using axial x-rays. May be performed with or without iodinated contrast. Provides clear pictures of both bone and soft tissues. Ideal for identifying hemorrhage or signs of trauma.

MRI

Magnetic resonance imaging creates computer-generated images using magnets instead of x-rays. May be performed with or without gadolinium contrast. Provides clear pictures of fluids and brain structures but not bone. May be used for identifying brain or vascular pathology in non-emergent, non-traumatic headaches.

Chapter 3

Term

Migraine symptoms

Aura

Definition

Focal neurological symptoms that precede the painful part of migraine in some patients. Usually visual change or numbness.

Allodynia

Perception of pain after receiving a skin stimulus that is not ordinarily painful (such as light touch).

Prodrome

Premonitory symptoms that occur several hours to days before the painful stage of migraine.

Postdrome

Residual discomfort that persists after the painful stage of migraine has resolved.

Scotoma	Characteristic aura symptoms described as blind spots in the visual field.
Teichopsia	Characteristic aura symptoms described as zigzag lines.

Pediatric migraine variants

Abdominal migraine	Episodes of midline abdominal pain without gastrointestinal disease in school-aged children.
Acute confusional state	Periods of short duration delirium in older children.
Benign paroxysmal vertigo	Intermittent, brief periods of marked imbalance in pre-school age children.
Benign paroxysmal torticollis	Episodic, involuntary head tilting or turning in infants and toddlers.
Cyclic vomiting	Recurring bouts of vomiting without identified gastrointestinal disease in infants and young children.

Chapter 4

Term	**Definition**
Cortical spreading depression	A slowly progressive wave across the cortex of initial neuronal excitation, followed by reduced activity, is believed to cause migraine aura.
Hyperexcitability	Enhanced activation within the brain, postulated to be the physiological basis for migraine.

Serotonin	A neurotransmitter found in blood platelets, the digestive system, and the brain. Also called 5-hydroxytryptamine or 5HT.
Trigeminal	Related to the fifth cranial nerve, a major relay station for pain from the head and face.
Up-regulation	Increase in number of receptors, leading to increased sensitivity.

Chapter 5

Term	**Definition**
Acute treatment	Treatment designed to reduce the severity of a current headache episode. Previously called *abortive* treatment.
Preventive	Treatment designed to reduce the frequency or severity of future headache episodes. Previously called *prophylactic* treatment.
Pain-free response	Reduction in headache pain to no pain.
Relief	Reduction in headache severity to no or mild symptoms.
Sustained relief	Headache relief with no increase in severity of headache symptoms during the first 24 hours after initial improvement.

Chapter 6

Term	Definition
Co-occurring	Conditions that occur in the same patient by chance alone or coincidence. May also be called *co-existing*.
Comorbid	One disease or disorder occurs at the same time as a separate disorder. Although these conditions represent two unique conditions, they occur together more frequently than would be expected by chance occurrence.
Hazard ratio	Estimates relative risk using a survival analysis.
Odds ratio	Method for comparing the probability of conditions occurring together.
Relative risk	Risk of an event in one group divided by the risk of that same event in a comparator, control group.

Chapter 7

Term	Definition
Acupuncture	Technique for inserting thin needles into the skin at specific body regions and stimulating these points to reduce symptoms.
Alternative medicine	Therapies designed to replace traditional medical treatment.
Biofeedback	A relaxation technique that uses external monitors to help identify when an appropriate relaxation response has been achieved.

Botulinum toxin or botox	Botulinum toxin A produced by *Clostridium botulinum* and injected in small amounts into muscles to achieve a temporary, localized paralysis.
Complementary medicine	Therapies designed to supplement traditional medical treatment.
Relaxation	A state of reduced physiological excitation achieved by using specific techniques.

Chapter 8

Term	**Definition**
Adolescence	Period between puberty and adulthood.
Adolescent	Persons ages 12-17 years old.
Child	Persons <12 years old.
Menopause	Portion of the female lifecycle after menstruation has permanently ceased.
Perimenopause	Time of transition, usually about six months before menopause. During this time, hormone levels fluctuate, resulting in menstrual irregularities, hot flashes, sweating, and other somatic symptoms.
Postmenopause	The time after menstrual periods have been absent for 12 consecutive months, with no other explanation for this change.

Chapter 9

Term	Definition
Anti-emetic	Treatment primarily designed to reduce nausea, usually by inhibiting dopamine activity.
Glascow Coma Scale	Standard severity measure of acute brain injury. Described in detail in Chapter 2.
Headache-specific treatment	Medications whose primary indication is headache relief. Includes dihydro-ergotamine and triptans.
Recurrence	Usually refers to the return of headache symptoms within 24 hours after initial successful treatment.

Chapter 10

Term	Definition
Arteritis	Inflammatory condition affecting arteries.
Basilar	Symptoms may be related to the brainstem functions.
Dysphasia	Disturbance of reception and/or expression of verbal or written speech. Severe dysphasia produces aphasia, an inability to understand or produce speech.
Hemicrania	Affecting either the left or right side of the head.
Hemiplegic	Marked weakness or paralysis affecting either the right or left side of the body.
Hypnic	Related to sleep.

Neuralgia	Intense pain caused by nerve irritation or injury, usually perceived as burning or electrical.
Neuropathic treatment	Antidepressants and anti-epileptic medications offer good reduction in pain related to nerve injury or irritation.
Paroxysmal	Sudden, recurrent attacks.
Pseudotumor cerebri	Previously used term to describe condition of increased intracranial pressure in the absence of causative inflammatory, structural, or mass lesions.
Shingles	Acute, painful infection with blistering skin lesions in a dermatomal distribution caused by herpes zoster, occurring after exposure to chicken pox or reactivation of herpes zoster virus.
Transient visual obscurations	Temporary blindness typically lasting <1 minute associated with increased intracranial pressure. Characteristically occurs when rising from sitting to standing position.
Trigeminal	Relating to the fifth cranial nerve, which functions to supply sensation to the face and motor function to the muscles of mastication.

About the author

Dawn Marcus is a diplomate of the American Board of Neurology and Psychiatry. Since 1990, she has been a faculty member at the University of Pittsburgh Medical Center, and is currently a professor in the Department of Anesthesiology. She has treated patients with a variety of chronic pain complaints at the Pain Evaluation and Treatment Institute at the University of Pittsburgh. She is also the Director of Research at the Multidisciplinary Headache Clinic.

Dr. Marcus has authored over 100 articles on the topics of chronic pain and headache, and has given numerous training sessions and invited lectures on the topics of chronic pain and headache in the United States and internationally. She has also been the principal investigator on research projects investigating pain epidemiology, pathology, treatment, and women's issues that have been funded by regional or national sources. She is the author of six books on chronic pain and migraine for both the professional and lay readerships, and in 2007 Dr Marcus won the Excellence in Media Award from the National Headache Foundation.

Acknowledgements

I would like to acknowledge the following for their help in supplying the front cover images:

Left: Medulloblastoma in a child with new onset, occipital headache, blurred vision, and balance disturbance.

Courtesy of Clayton A. Wiley, MD/PhD, Professor, Department of Pathology, Neuropathology, University of Pittsburgh.

Centre: Non-specific white spots commonly seen in migraine patients.
Right: Arnold Chiari malformation with hydrocephalus.
Background: Papilledema.

Courtesy of Rock A. Heyman, MD, Assistant Professor of Neurology, University of Pittsburgh Medical Center.

Chapter 1

Epidemiology of headache

Introduction

Pain is the number one somatic complaint seen in ambulatory care (Figure 1) [1]. Back pain is the most common complaint (10%), followed by lower extremity pain (9%), and upper extremity pain and headache (each 6%). Similarly, the National Health and Nutrition Examination Survey

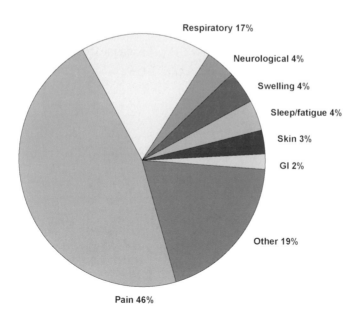

Figure 1 Somatic complaints in primary care office visits. GI includes gastroenteritis and nausea. (Based on Khan 2003.)

reported active, problematic localized chronic pain with episodes lasting at least 24 hours in an estimated 11% of adults in the United States, with chronic widespread pain in 4% of adults [2]. This survey only included reports of major pain, resulting in a substantially lower prevalence of headache pain than reported in the studies cited in the next section, which included any headache complaint. Head pain was the fourth most common individual pain location (Figure 2), with head pain more common among women and variability within genders based on race (Figure 3).

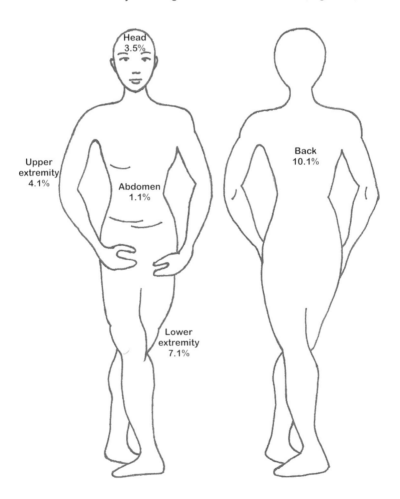

Head
3.5%

Upper
extremity
4.1%

Abdomen
1.1%

Back
10.1%

Lower
extremity
7.1%

Figure 2 Estimated prevalence of major chronic pain with episodes lasting ≥24 hours by body regions. (Based on Hardt 2008.)

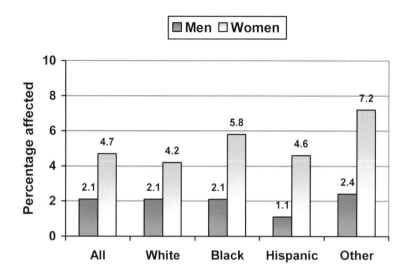

Figure 3 Gender and ethnic differences in major head pain population prevalence estimates. (Based on Hardt 2008.)

Headache epidemiology

Headache is endorsed as a current complaint by nearly half of all adults worldwide (Figure 4), with two in every three adults affected at some point during their lives [3]. The vast majority of chronic headache patients are managed by primary care physicians (PCPs). According to the National Ambulatory Medical Care Survey, two in every three migraine patients are treated by PCPs, with only 17% treated by neurologists [4].

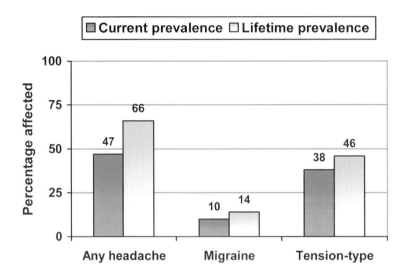

Figure 4 Worldwide headache prevalence. (Based on Stovner 2007.)

Acute or new onset headaches may be caused by systemic illness, such as infection or intracranial pathology (Table 1). Head pain may also occur as a consequence of musculoskeletal dysfunction in the neck or cervical spine. Chronic headache is most commonly caused by primary headache disorders, although some secondary headaches (like post-trauma headache, trigeminal neuralgia, post-herpetic neuralgia, and analgesic overuse headache) may also result in chronic pain syndromes.

Table 1 Common causes of head pain.

Primary headaches
- Migraine
- Tension-type
- Cluster

Secondary headaches
- Infection
  - Viral illness
  - Respiratory infection
  - Meningitis

- Inflammatory
  - Giant cell arteritis
  - Systemic lupus erythematosus

- Intracranial pathology
  - Cerebrovascular disease
  - Subdural hematoma
  - Tumor
  - Vascular malformation or aneurysm

- Medications
  - Analgesic overuse headache
  - Alcohol-induced headache
  - Caffeine, opioid, or estrogen withdrawal

- Musculoskeletal
  - Temporomandibular dysfunction
  - Cervical myofascial or joint dysfunction

- Neuralgias
  - Post-herpetic neuralgia
  - Trigeminal neuralgia

- Systemic illness
  - Anemia
  - Thyroid disease

Adult headaches

Acute headaches

Patients with new onset acute or a recent change in headache will require a more thorough evaluation to rule out secondary conditions than patients with stable, chronic headaches. Patients reporting new headaches often experience headaches related to an acute viral illness or trauma.

Headaches seen in the emergency department (ED) may be acute headaches or recalcitrant chronic headaches. In most cases, non-traumatic head pain conditions seen in the ED are caused by primary, recurring headaches. In a prospective, observational survey, discharge diagnoses were analyzed for all patients presenting to an ED with a chief complaint of non-traumatic headache over 11 months [5]. Migraine was the most common individual diagnosis (Table 2). A pathological diagnosis is most common among older ED patients. Using data from the National Hospital Ambulatory Medical Care Survey, a pathological headache (including meningitis, encephalitis, stroke, hemorrhage, aneurysm, glaucoma, benign intracranial hypertension, giant cell/temporal arteritis, or hypertensive encephalopathy) accounted for 2% of non-traumatic headaches in all ED patients, 6% of non-traumatic headaches in patients ≥50 years old and 11% in those ≥75 years old [6].

Chronic headaches

The most common types of chronically recurring headaches are tension-type and migraine. Patients with chronic headache, like migraine or tension-type headache, who overuse pain medications may develop a second type of headache, called medication overuse headache. Post-trauma and cluster headaches are less common.

Table 2 Discharge diagnoses in consecutive ED patients with non-traumatic headache. (Based on Fiesseler 2005.)

Diagnosis	Percentage
Migraine	41
Undifferentiated	37
Infection	10
Tension-type headache	4
Cluster headache	2
Stroke, transient ischemic attack, intracranial hemorrhage	2
Post-lumbar puncture headache	2
Benign intracranial hypertension (pseudotumor cerebri)	1
Glaucoma	1

Migraine and tension-type headaches

Migraine is an intermittent, disabling headache (Table 3), while tension-type headache is a milder headache that does not typically limit activities (Table 4). In community samples of adults recording active headache, tension-type headache affects nearly four times as many people as migraine (Figure 5) [3]. Although tension-type headache is more prevalent than migraine, migraineurs are more likely to seek care [7]. Consequently, most patients seen in primary care for chronic, recurring headaches have migraine. An international survey of primary care patients seeking treatment for headache revealed a diagnosis of migraine in 94%, with tension-type headache in only 3% (Figure 5) [8].

Table 3 Migraine.

- Intermittent moderate-severe headache

- Typical duration = 8-24 hours

- Disabling headache that limits activities

- Pain is often throbbing

- Pain often affects one side of the head

- Pain accompanied by sensitivity to lights and noise or nausea

- Patient characteristically seeks quiet isolation

- Typically familial

- Often worse with menstrual period

- Visual disturbance or hallucinations (aura) precedes or accompanies headache for 25% of patients

Table 4 Tension-type.

- Constant or intermittent mild-moderate headache

- May last hours to days

- Does not interfere with activity

- Often described as a squeezing band across forehead

- Generally not associated with sensitivity to lights and noise or nausea

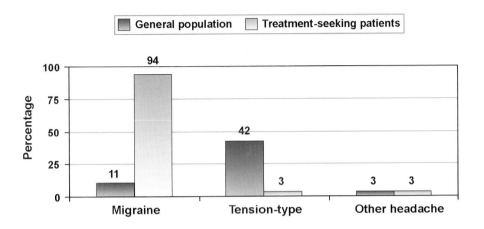

Figure 5 Prevalence of active headache in general population and treatment-seeking primary care patient samples. (Based on Tepper 2004, Stovner 2007.)

Medication overuse headache

Medication overuse headaches occur as a reaction to excessive analgesic or headache medication use and affect 0.5-1% of adults worldwide [3]. Daily or near daily use of medications designed to treat individual headache episodes can result in a change and worsening of underlying headache if used regularly for at least six weeks. Medication overuse headache is typically a mild, bilateral, pressure headache with fluctuating severity (Table 5). Patients with medication overuse headache often experience daily mild, bilateral headaches plus intermittent, severe migraines.

Table 5 Medication overuse headache.

- Daily or constant headache

- Pain often affects both sides of the head

- Pain may vary from mild-severe. Usually not disabling

- Patient diary characteristically reveals using repeated daily doses of analgesics and/or headache relief medications

Medication overuse headache typically occurs in patients with a primary complaint of frequent migraine, tension-type, or post-trauma headache, who begin overusing headache remedies. Both analgesics and migraine-specific relieving medications (e.g., ergotamines or triptans) may contribute to medication overuse headache. A recent survey identified acetaminophen, non-steroidal anti-inflammatory drugs, triptans and butalbital as the most common culprits of medication overuse headache (Figure 6) [9]. Low-dose

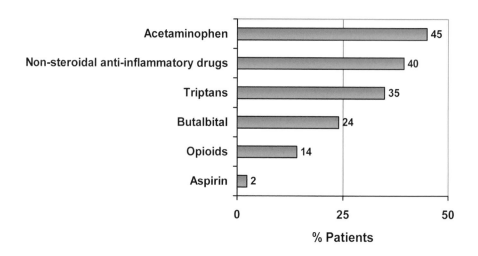

Figure 6 Medications associated with medication overuse headache. (Based on Meskunas 2006.)

aspirin for a cardioprotective effect does not result in medication overuse headache. Probable medication overuse headache should be considered in patients with benign headache taking an individual drug or combination of medications on a regular basis three or more days per week. Switching among different drugs designed to treat individual headache episodes on different days does not minimize the risk of medication overuse headache.

Post-trauma headache

Chronic headache may also begin as a consequence of mild head injury (Table 6). Post-trauma headache begins within seven days of a mild head injury associated with concussion. A concussion should be diagnosed when patients have any of the following symptoms following head trauma: "feel dazed," "see stars," have amnesia for events before or after the accident, or experience a brief loss of consciousness. Post-concussive syndrome features often accompany post-traumatic headaches and may include: depressed or irritable mood, memory loss, dizziness or vertigo, and tinnitus. A survey of 357 college athletes who had sustained sport-related concussions revealed headache in 70% of football players and 73% of soccer players [10]. Post-trauma headache is more likely to occur after a motor vehicle accident when whiplash has occurred (22% with whiplash vs. 7% without whiplash) [11].

Table 6 Post-trauma.

- Headache occurs within 1 week of mild concussion

- Patient will describe "seeing stars," "feeling dazed," loss of consciousness <30 minutes, or amnesia with head injury

- Initial headache is often severe, disabling, and constant

- After 2 months, headache usually becomes milder and intermittent

- Typically resolves after 3-12 months

- May be accompanied by dizziness, mood disturbance or irritability, or cognitive impairment

a

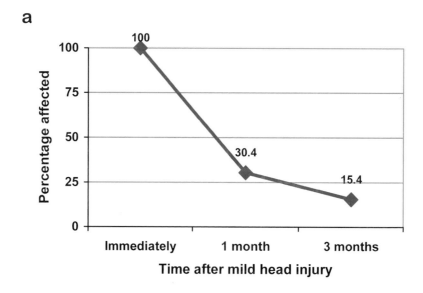

b

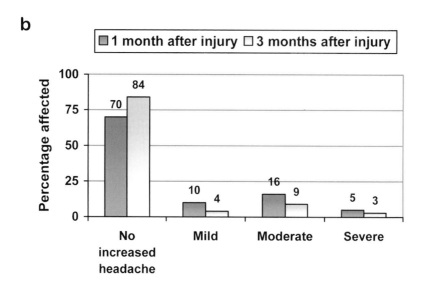

Figure 7 Natural history of post-trauma headaches. a) Prevalence over time. b) Severity over time (no increased headache means headache-free or headache returned to pre-injury pattern). (Based on Faux 2007.)

Pain is often constant and severe immediately after mild head injury. Post-traumatic headache should improve from constant and severe to milder and less frequent over the first two weeks. Headaches failing to improve, worsening, or associated with progressive post-concussive symptoms should be re-evaluated with imaging studies to rule out subacute pathology, such as a subdural hematoma or an undiagnosed fracture. Headache features are often consistent with migraine in the early phases of post-trauma headache, and become milder like tension-type headache when post-trauma headache persists. Post-trauma headache resolves within one month for every two of three patients (Figure 7) [12]. In those patients with persisting post-trauma headaches, the pain tends to become more intermittent and less severe.

Cluster headache

Cluster headache is an intermittent headache, experienced as brief, recurring episodes of excruciating, peri-orbital pain (Table 7). These headaches tend to occur in groups or clusters occurring once or twice yearly and typically lasting about six weeks. During a cluster, patients usually experience one to four headache episodes nightly. Between clusters, patients are generally headache-free. Autonomic features of marked lacrimation and rhinorrhea are often touted as pathognomonic for cluster headache, although few patients endorse these symptoms, probably due to the extreme pain severity.

Table 7 Cluster.

- Intermittent, short duration, very severe headache

- Typical duration = 30-90 minutes

- Generally attacks occur at night

- Pain typically affects one eye/peri-orbital area

- Patient often smokes, paces, or showers during attacks

- Patient may bang head during attack

- Observer may notice lacrimation and rhinorrhea

Cluster headache is relatively uncommon, occurring in <1% of adults. The incidence of cluster headache has decreased markedly over the last several decades. The overall incidence rate in Rochester, Minnesota, during 1979-1981 was 10 cases per 100,000 persons, dropping to 2 per 100,000 between 1989-1990 [13]. Furthermore, the male predominance of cluster has also decreased in recent decades, with a 6:1 male predominance reported during the 1960s decreasing to a 2:1 predominance in the 1990s [14]. Changes in lifestyle, such as increased female use of alcohol and tobacco, as well as the increased role of women in the workforce, have been postulated to contribute to this changing epidemiology.

Women's headaches

When tested with experimental pain, women have a lower pain threshold and pain tolerance than men, resulting in increased sensitivity to painful stimuli [15]. Women tend to perceive painful signals earlier and more acutely than their male counterparts. This increased sensitivity to pain may explain the increased prevalence of many painful conditions, including headache, in women. Most common recurring headaches occur more frequently in women (Table 8).

Table 8 Headache prevalence ratios comparing genders.

Headache diagnosis	Males	Females
Migraine	1	3
Tension-type	1	2
Post-trauma	1	2
Cluster	2	1

Predictable changes in headache, especially migraine, occur in females in relation to changing levels of estrogen (Table 9) [16]. Estrogen acts as an important pain modulator. Cycling estradiol often precipitates headache onset and subsequent aggravation of headache. Increasing estrogen levels (e.g., during pregnancy) and discontinuation of cycling (e.g., after menopause) offer a headache protective effect.

Table 9 Changes in primary headache in women.

Reproductive status	Migraine pattern
Menarche	Onset of migraine
Menses	Aggravation for 60% of women
Oral contraceptive use	Migraine typically aggravated during placebo week
Pregnancy	Migraine relief in 50-80% during 2nd and 3rd trimesters Headaches generally return after delivery Breastfeeding may delay migraine return
Menopause	Aggravation typical during perimenopause Migraine improves in 2 of 3 postmenopausal women

Geriatric headache

New-onset headache or head pain in seniors should be evaluated for possible secondary headaches as primary headaches typically do not begin after age 50. Commonly occurring secondary headaches may include headaches related to cervical disease (e.g., arthritis), giant cell (temporal) arteritis, trigeminal neuralgia, post-herpetic neuralgia, or intracranial pathology. A more complete description of geriatric headaches is provided in Chapter 10.

Recurring headaches during the preceding year are reported by one in five seniors (26% of women and 16% of men) [17]. Migraine prevalence decreases in seniors, while tension-type headaches persist (Figure 8) [18].

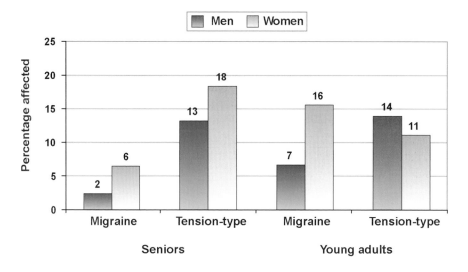

Figure 8 Prevalence of recurring headache in seniors (mean age = 75 years) and young adults (mean age = 22 years). (Based on Camarda 2003 and Deleu 2001.)

Headache-related disability

The World Health Organization has identified migraine among the top 20 causes of disability worldwide, ranking 12th for women and 19th for both genders combined [19]. Three in every four employed adult migraineurs experience lost time from work due to migraine, with an average loss of 4.4 days annually [20]. Family and social relationships are also substantially affected by migraine (Table 10) [21].

Table 10 Migraine-related disability. (Based on Lipton 2003.)

Disability	Percentage
Avoided planning family or social activities	32
Missed family or social activities ≥3 days during previous 3 months	19
Moderate to marked decrease in household chores	85
Moderate to marked negative impact on relationship with child(ren)	63
Migraineur's child missed school or was tardy due to parent's migraine	19

Headache comorbidity

The National Comorbidity Survey Replication evaluated the presence of comorbid illnesses in adults with migraine (N=317), non-migraine headache (N=400), or no headache (N=4767) [22]. Both physical and psychological illnesses occur significantly more often in headache sufferers (Table 11). Common comorbidities are other chronic pain conditions (especially arthritis and back or neck pain), anxiety, mood disturbance, and hypertension.

Table 11 Headache comorbidity. Prevalence of comorbid conditions and odds ratios, based on presence of headache. (Based on Saunders 2008.)

Condition	Prevalence based on headache (%)			Odds ratio	
	Migraine	Non-migraine	No headache	Migraine vs. no headache	Non-migraine vs. no headache
Any comorbidity	82.5	78.5	50.8	3.5*	2.8*
Physical comorbidity					
Any	46.6	44.2	38.7	2.1*	1.7*
Chronic non-headache pain	58.3	57.8	36.3	3.3*	3.5*
Hypertension	20.5	16.1	19.2	2.1*	1.2
Irritable bowel	3.7	1.5	0.7	3.8*	1.8
Peptic ulcer	5.7	4.6	2.0	2.5*	2.4*
Mental comorbidity					
Any	53.1	38.0	20.8	3.1*	2.0*
Mood disorder	24.7	17.5	6.7	3.2*	2.5*
Anxiety disorder	44.5	30.9	15.5	3.1*	2.0*

* Odds ratio is significant at $P \leq 0.05$.

Pediatric headache

Acute headaches

Similar to adults, headaches presenting to the ED in children and adolescents are commonly caused by infection, trauma, or a primary headache disorder. In a recent survey of pediatric ED patients with non-traumatic headache, most patients had a primary headache diagnosis, with migraine diagnosed in 10% of primary headache patients (Figure 9) [23]. Acute viral and respiratory infection accounted for 91% of secondary headaches. Pathological diagnoses occurred in only 4% of patients, including neurological conditions (e.g., seizures, vestibular neuritis, shunt malfunction, cerebrovascular conditions, meningitis, and tumors), carbon monoxide intoxication, and hypertension. All patients with neurological conditions had pathological findings in their history (e.g., loss of consciousness or focal deficits) or physical examination.

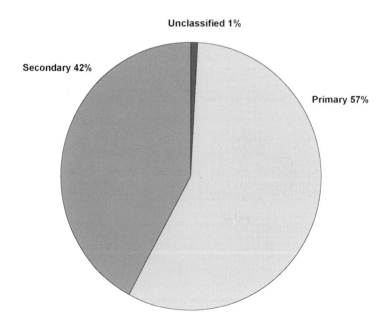

Figure 9 ED diagnoses in pediatric patients with headache. (Based on Scagni 2008.)

Chronic headaches

Recurring headaches are commonly reported in children and adolescents, with headaches often continuing into adulthood. A prospective diary study of 2126 children aged 7-12 years identified any headache during the preceding month in 58% of children, with frequent headache in one in ten children [24]. Headaches become more prevalent during adolescence. A community survey reported headache in the preceding six months in 53% of children surveyed, with any headache and migraine more common in adolescents (Figure 10) [25]. The mean age at headache onset was 7.5 years, with 5% of children reporting headache onset at age three or younger. Headache onset was earlier in boys than girls (7.3 vs. 7.8 years, P<0.001). Headache duration was shorter in children than adults, with headache episodes lasting ≤2 hours for 59% of children.

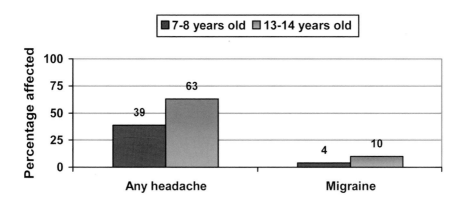

Figure 10 Prevalence of pediatric headache. (Kröner-Herwig 2007.)

Childhood headache is important because children with headache lose an average of 7.8 days per school year, compared with 3.7 days per year lost for children without headaches [26]. Frequent school absenteeism is a significant stressor, resulting in loss of academic performance, social interaction with peers, and self-esteem. These factors, themselves, often aggravate pain perception. Although children and adolescents rarely identify school stress as a headache trigger, pediatric headaches characteristically occur on school days (Figure 11) [27], most commonly on Monday through Wednesday between 6 AM to 6 PM [28]. The strong influence of school stress on pediatric migraine often leads to the false interpretation by peers, teachers, and parents that pediatric headaches are fictitious excuses to avoid schoolwork rather than a physiological reaction to school-related stressors.

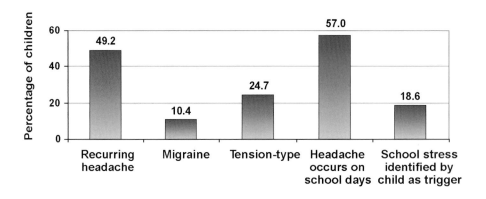

Figure 11 Prevalence of recurring headache and relation to school in 8-16-year-old children. (Based on Ozge 2003.)

Conclusions

Headaches affect about half of all children and adults, representing one of the most common complaints seen in primary care. Most non-traumatic headaches for which patients seek treatment can be diagnosed as migraine. Chronic headaches substantially impair work productivity, social activities, and family relationships. Furthermore, migraine sufferers are three times more likely to also experience a comorbid psychological or physical illness in comparison with non-headache individuals. The high prevalence and significant negative impact from chronic headache conditions suggest a need for effective identification and management of headache complaints in clinical practice.

Key Summary

◆ Headache is the fourth most common somatic complaint seen in primary care.

◆ About half of adults and children report active headache.

◆ Most non-traumatic headaches seen by primary care practitioners are primary headaches, especially migraine.

◆ Women's headaches change with reproductive status, with increased headache activity with estrogen cycling and decreased headache with elevated estradiol.

◆ New-onset headaches in seniors are often secondary headaches.

◆ Chronic headaches result in substantial loss of school and work time, as well as social and family impairments.

◆ Common migraine comorbidities include other chronic pain, mood disturbance, and hypertension.

References

1. Khan AA, Khan A, Harezlak J, Tu W, Kroenke K. Somatic symptoms in primary care: etiology and outcome. *Psychosomatics* 2003; 44: 471-478.
2. Hardt J, Jacobsen C, Goldberg J, Nickel R, Buchwald D. Prevalence of chronic pain in a representative sample in the United States. *Pain Medicine*, in press.
3. Stovner LJ, Hagen K, Jensen R, *et al.* The global burden of headache: a documentation of headache prevalence and disability worldwide. *Cephalalgia* 2007; 27: 193-210.
4. Gibbs TS, Fleischer AB, Feldman SR, Sam MC, O'Donovan CA. Health care utilization in patients with migraine: demographics and patterns of care in the ambulatory setting. *Headache* 2003; 43: 330-335.
5. Fiesseler FW, Riggs RL, Holubek W, Eskin B, Richman PB. Canadian Headache Society criteria for the diagnosis of acute migraine headache in the ED - do our patients meet these criteria? *Am J Emerg Med* 2005; 23: 149-154.
6. Goldstein JN, Camargo CA, Pelletier AJ, Edlow JA. Headache in the United States emergency departments: demographics, work-up and frequency of pathological disease. *Cephalalgia* 2006; 26: 684-690.
7. Hasse LA, Ritchey N, Smith R. Predicting the number of headache visits by type of patient seen in family practice. *Headache* 2002; 42: 738-746.
8. Tepper SJ, Dahlöf CH, Dowson A, *et al.* Prevalence and diagnosis of migraine in patients consulting their physician with a complaint of headache: data from the Landmark study. *Headache* 2004; 44: 856-864.
9. Meskunas CA, Tepper SJ, Rapoport AM, Sheftell FD. Medications associated with probable medication overuse headache reported in a tertiary care headache center over a 15-year period. *Headache* 2006; 46: 766-772.
10. Delaney JS, Lacroix VJ, Leclerc S, Johnston KM. Concussions among university football and soccer players. *Clin J Sport Med* 2002; 12: 331-338.
11. Berglund A, Alfredsson L, Jensen I, Cassidy JD, Nygren A. The association between exposure to a rear-end collision and future health complaints. *J Clin Epidemiol* 2001; 54: 851-856.
12. Faux S, Sheedy J. A prospective controlled study in the prevalence of posttraumatic headache following mild traumatic brain injury. *Pain Medicine*, in press.
13. Black DF, Swanson JW, Stang PE. Decreasing incidence of cluster headache: a population-based study in Olmsted County, Minnesota. *Headache* 2005; 45: 220-223.
14. Manzoni GC. Gender ratio of cluster headache over the years: a possible role of changes in lifestyle. *Cephalalgia* 1998; 18: 138-142.
15. Walker JS, Carmody JJ. Experimental pain in healthy human subjects: gender differences in nociception and in response to ibuprofen. *Anesth Analg* 1998; 86: 1257-1262.
16. Loder E, Marcus DA. *Migraine in Women*. BC Decker: London, Ontario, 2003.
17. Camarda R, Monastero R. Prevalence of primary headaches in Italian elderly: preliminary data from the Zabút Aging Project. *Neurol Sci* 2003; 24: S122-S124.
18. Deleu D, Khan MA, Humaidan H, Al Mantheri Z, Al Hashami S. Prevalence and clinical characteristics of headache in medical students in Oman. *Headache* 2001; 41: 798-804.

19. Leonardi M, Steiner TJ, Scher AT, Lipton RB. The global burden of migraine: measuring disability in headache disorders with WHO's Classification of Functioning, Disability and Health (ICF). *J Headache Pain* 2005; 6: 429-440.

20. Lofland JH, Frick KD. Workplace absenteeism and aspects of access to health care for individuals with migraine. *Headache* 2006; 46: 563-576.

21. Lipton RB, Bigal ME, Kolodner K, *et al.* The family impact of migraine: population-based studies in the USA and UK. *Cephalalgia* 2003; 23: 429-440.

22. Saunders K, Merikangas K, Low NP, Von Korff M, Kessler RC. Impact of comorbidity on headache-related disability. *Neurology* 2008; 70: 538-547.

23. Scagni P, Pagliero R. Headache in an Italian pediatric emergency department. *J Headache Pain* 2008; 9: 83-87.

24. Lundqvist C, Clench-Aas J, Hofoss D, Bartonova A. Self-reported headache in schoolchildren: parents underestimate their children's headaches. *Acta Pediatrica* 2006; 95: 940-946.

25. Kröner-Herwig B, Heinrich M, Morris L. Headache in German children and adolescents: a population-based epidemiological study. *Cephalalgia* 2007; 27: 519-527.

26. Abu-Arafeh I, Russell G. Prevalence of headache and migraine in schoolchildren. *Br Med J* 1994; 309: 765-769.

27. Ozge A, Bugdayci R, Sasmaz T, *et al.* The sensitivity and specificity of the case definition criteria in diagnosis of headache: a school-based epidemiological study of 5562 children in Mersin. *Cephalalgia* 2003; 23: 138-145.

28. Winner P, Putnam G, Saiers J, O'Quinn S, Asgharnejad M. Demographic and migraine characteristics of adolescent patients: the Glaxo Wellcome adolescent clinical trials database. *Headache* 2000; 40: 438.

Chapter 2

Diagnostic testing in the headache patient

Introduction

The diagnostic work-up of headaches may include:

◆ history;
◆ physical examination;
◆ specialized testing.

As with most medical conditions, the majority of details gathered to help determine the cause and best treatment for headache occurs through collecting a comprehensive analysis of historical information. Physical examination findings may occasionally uncover unexpected pathology, although both physical examination and specialized testing generally confirm or refute diagnoses anticipated from a careful history.

Headache history

Patients presenting with a complaint of headache or change in headache pattern should be questioned about their general health as well as headache activity. A series of questions can be used to help determine both the likely preliminary diagnosis or diagnoses and the need for additional testing (Table 1). Always ask patients to identify how many different types of headaches they have. If they have more than one headache, ask them to answer questions for their most severe and their mildest headache separately. Often patients who report >2 different

Table 1 Headache history questionnaire.

Question	Response
How many types of headache do you have?	If >1, answer the questions below separately for the most severe and the mildest headache.
How long have your headaches been the way they are now?	Additional testing (e.g., imaging studies) may be needed if headaches are new or have changed within the last 2 years.
How often do you get a headache? Do you have days without any headache?	Ask about possible medication overuse in patients reporting headaches >3 days per week. Patients with headaches usually occurring >3 days per week will need to focus on prevention therapy.
How long does each headache last?	Most headaches last 8-12 hours. Short duration headaches (<2 hours) may be cluster headache. Headaches lasting >12 hours may need a medication of longer duration.
What do you typically do when you get a headache? Are you able to continue your regular activities or do you need to restrict activities?	Patients with tension-type headache generally continue their activities, while those with migraine often retreat to dark, quiet isolation (due to photophobia and phonophobia). Sleeping often relieves a migraine. Disabling chronic headache is usually a migraine. Cluster patients conversely become very active during an attack, pacing, smoking, showering, or banging their heads.
Do you get sick to your stomach with your headache?	Patients with tension-type headache may lose their appetites, but are generally not nauseated. Migraineurs are often nauseated, and vomiting characteristically reduces migraine symptoms.
Are you having your typical headache right now? If so, is this as severe as it typically gets?	Directly observe patient behaviors to judge interference with activities and sensitivity to conversational speech and room lighting in patients experiencing typical headache during the visit.

Table 1 Headache history questionnaire *continued.*

Question	Response
Where do you get your pain? Is the pain ALWAYS in the same spot or does it sometimes change sides of the head?	The location of tension-type headache is often variable. Cluster headache is generally always around the same eye with every episode. Migraine may usually be on one side of the head, but it will typically occasionally affect the other side. Migraine always affecting the same location will need additional work-up, such as imaging studies to rule out underlying pathology, e.g., an arteriovenous malformation.
Have you developed any other health problems since your headaches began or changed?	Patients with additional medical or neurological complaints will need a more extensive work-up.
Have you found a pattern for when your headaches occur or get worse?	Patients may be suspicious of certain triggers. Completing a daily headache-recording diary (see below) can confirm or uncover important patterns.
What medications do you take? What do you take when you get a headache? How about over-the-counter medications? How about herbs or nutritional supplements? Have you recently changed your medications?	Headache is a common side effect of medications. Patients using excessive amounts of pain or headache-relieving medications may have medication overuse headache. Understanding all of the drugs used by your patient (including over-the-counter and nutritional) is essential for safe prescribing.

headaches have only one or two unique types of headache, with differences in severity incorrectly identified as separate headache disorders.

Diary collection

Reviewing prospectively collected headache information supplements information supplied during history taking. Daily headache diaries are excellent tools for collecting information about headache and medication use patterns that may not be readily recognized by patient recall alone.

Asking patients to log headache severity several times daily helps provide important information about headache duration and pain severity fluctuation. A sample diary is provided in Figure 1.

Name: _____

Date: _____/_____/_____

Time of day	Severity				Medications
	None	Mild	Moderate	Severe	
Morning					
Noon					
Evening					
Bedtime					

List possible triggers:

Did you have your menstrual period today?   Circle   YES   NO

Figure 1 Daily headache diary.

Daily headache recordings should be collected for one to two months in all new headache patients to help identify a correct diagnosis and determine the most appropriate therapy. Diaries are also useful when headache patterns change and to monitor response to treatment interventions.

Physical examination

The physical examination of the headache patient should include inspection of the head, as well as thorough general medical, neurological, and musculoskeletal evaluations (Table 2). Patients with limitations on

Table 2 Headache physical examination.

Examination	Interpretation
General examination	
Vital signs	Fever suggests infection. Elevated blood pressure may also contribute to head pain.
Inspection of the head	Rarely produces positive findings, but builds confidence with the patient who may be upset if you never directly examine the body part with pain.
Neurologic examination	
Cranial nerves • Fundoscopy • Eye movements • Facial symmetry	Papilledema suggests increased intracranial pressure. Patients with abnormal eye movements or unexplained facial asymmetry may require additional testing.
Gait	Both sides of the body should move in a similar fashion with casual walking. Patients with an abnormal gait will need a more detailed neurological exam.
Strength and reflexes	Look for patterns of weakness and motor loss that suggest focal deficits, radiculopathy, or other specific neurological condition.
Sensation	Look for patterns of numbness that suggest focal deficits, radiculopathy, neuropathy, or other specific neurological condition.
Musculoskeletal	
Resting posture and range of motion	Abnormal posture or range of motion may suggest dysfunction or pathology in the neck muscles or cervical spine that can produce or aggravate head pain. These patients may need additional radiographic testing.
Palpation	Tender areas on the posterior head or neck that may aggravate head pain suggest possible occipital neuralgia or myofascial pain that may respond to injections and physical therapy treatments.

active range of motion will need additional passive testing with the patient relaxed. A musculoskeletal examination of the neck can be limited in patients with neck pain or anxiety, due to excessive pain, muscle spasm, or co-contraction of opposing muscle groups restricting range of motion assessment. A physical therapy evaluation may be necessary to complete the musculoskeletal exam.

Specialized testing

Red flags

Supplemental testing (including blood tests, radiographic studies, or a spinal fluid examination) may be indicated in a patient whose history or examination suggests a secondary cause of headache. A variety of historical and examination findings provide red flags to suggest a greater possibility of a secondary headache disorder (Table 3). Any new headache, whether mild or severe, or change in headache pattern is important to assess.

Table 3 Red flags suggesting a need for additional work-up.

- Trauma

- Fever

- Seizures

- New headache

- Change in previously stable headache pattern

- History of malignancy

- Neurological symptoms or signs

- Patient ≥50 years of age

Laboratory testing

Blood tests are generally not indicated for patients with chronic headache. Blood tests may be recommended in patients with symptoms or signs suggesting additional medical conditions or in patients >50 years old to rule out giant cell arteritis (also called temporal arteritis) (Table 4).

Table 4 Recommended laboratory testing.

- Autoimmune tests (antinuclear antibody)

- Hematology (blood count)
  - Sedimentation rate or C-reactive protein and giant cell arteritis work-up for new headache in patients aged >50 years*

- Chemistries (electrolytes, liver and kidney function tests)

- Endocrine (thyroid function tests)

- Infectious (rapid plasma reagin for syphilis)

* See Chapter 10.

Radiographic imaging

In general, imaging studies are not recommended for patients with chronic headache unless patients have specific indications, and studies are being used to confirm or refute specific clinical diagnoses (Table 5). Indications would include joint abnormalities on examination, a new headache pattern, or abnormal neurological signs or symptoms, such as focal abnormalities, mental status changes, or seizures [1]. Magnetic resonance imaging (MRI) is preferred over computed tomography (CT) when brain imaging is recommended for non-emergent or non-traumatic headache. Unfortunately, clinically insignificant abnormalities occur with

Table 5 Recommended radiographic testing for chronic, non-traumatic headache.

Test	Indication	Interpretation caution
Brain MRI	New or changed headache, older patient age, neurological symptoms or signs	Non-specific white matter changes occur in 30% of migraineurs
Cervical spine x-ray	Abnormal posture, restricted range of motion, or pain reproduced with neck motion	False positives are common, especially in the lower cervical spine. Abnormalities occur in 1 in every 2-3 asymptomatic adults, especially at C5-6
Cervical spine MRI	Radiculopathy	False positives are common, especially in the lower cervical spine. Bulging discs may occur in up to 3 in every 4 asymptomatic adults, with herniated discs in half

MRI = magnetic resonance imaging

both plain x-rays and MRI scans in a substantial number of headache sufferers.

Plain x-rays of the cervical spine commonly show degenerative changes in adults. Radiographically-diagnosed degenerative cervical spine disease was determined in 159 asymptomatic adults (ages 20-65 years) at baseline and after ten years [2]. Lateral cervical spine x-ray abnormalities in the lower spine were seen in one in three patients at baseline and over half of patients when x-rays were repeated after ten years. Although only 15% of subjects experienced neck pain during the ensuing ten years, progressive degenerative changes were noted in 45% of subjects. The most commonly affected level was C5-6, although multilevel abnormalities were common. Degenerative changes on cervical spine x-rays are most prevalent with increased age, with abnormalities seen in 70% of women and 95% of men between the ages of 60-65 years old [3].

Similarly, clinically insignificant brain abnormalities on MRI occur in one in every three patients with migraine, most commonly non-specific white matter bright spots [4]. These false positives often lead to unnecessary anxiety about conditions like multiple sclerosis, cerebrovascular disease, or malignancy. In clinical experience, white spots may either resolve or persist when repeat imaging is conducted within six months. For this reason, routine imaging of chronic headache patients is discouraged. Insignificant abnormalities are also frequently identified with MRI of the cervical spine, with multiple level changes frequent among asymptomatic adults. In one survey, annular tears were identified in 37% of asymptomatic adults, with bulging discs in 73% and herniated discs in 50% [5]. Abnormalities most commonly affected the lower cervical levels, especially C5-6.

Spinal fluid assessment

A lumbar puncture is important in cases of suspected inflammatory disease (such as meningitis), subarachnoid hemorrhage, or benign intracranial hypertension. An imaging study of the head should be performed prior to lumbar puncture when:

◆ headache began after trauma;
◆ increased intracranial pressure or hemorrhage is suspected;
◆ a seizure has occurred;
◆ an altered level of consciousness or focal neurological signs are present.

Expected normal results from a lumbar puncture performed in the lateral recumbent position are given in Table 6 [6].

Table 6 Normal adult lumbar puncture results. (Based on Roos 2003.)

Test	Normal value
Opening pressure	180 mm H_2O (200-250 mm H_2O in obese patient)
White blood cells	0-5 mononuclear cells (lymphocytes and monocytes) 0 polymorphonuclear leukocytes
Glucose	65% of serum glucose <45mg/dL is abnormal
Protein	≤50mg/dL

Special circumstances

Evaluation after mild head injury

Patients reporting headache after trauma require additional testing to determine the severity and extent of injury. The Glasgow Coma Scale (GCS) is a routine measure of acute brain injury severity, with possible scores ranging from 3 to 15. Scores depend on patient responses, including eye opening and motor and verbal responses to stimulation (Table 7).

Table 7 Glasgow Coma Scale.

Eye opening		Best motor response		Best verbal response	
Action	*Score*	*Action*	*Score*	*Action*	*Score*
Spontaneous	4	Obeys verbal command	6	Oriented, converses	5
To speech	3	Localizes pain	5	Disoriented, converses	4
To pain	2	Flexion to pain - withdrawal	4	Inappropriate words	3
None	1	Flexion to pain - abnormal	3	Incomprehensible words	2
		Extension to pain	2	None	1
		None	1		

Sum of 3 scores=
Interpretation: Minor ≥13, Moderate 9-12, Severe ≤8

Post-trauma headache characteristically occurs after a mild head injury with concussion. Features defining a mild head injury are provided in Table 8. In addition to experiencing headache, patients often experience a variety of additional somatic and psychological complaints after trauma, called post-concussive syndrome, which occurs in 43% of patients experiencing a mild head injury (Table 9) [7].

Table 8 Definition of a mild head injury.

At least one of the following abnormalities	Severity
Loss of consciousness	≤30 minutes GCS after 30 minutes = 13-15
Memory loss for events immediately before or after trauma	≤24 hours after trauma
Abnormal mental state at the time of trauma	Feel dazed, disoriented, or confused
Focal neurological deficit	May be transient
GCS = Glasgow Coma Scale	

Table 9 Symptoms of post-concussive syndrome.

• Dizziness, vertigo, or tinnitus

• Fatigue or sleep disturbance

• Cognitive deficits (including attention, concentration, memory, or executive functions)

• Emotional irritability, emotional lability, or disinhibition

• Depression

A CT scan is the preferred imaging study in patients after trauma to identify blood and fractures. Studies of patients with mild head injury evaluated with CT identified abnormalities in 7-8% of patients [8, 9]. Factors associated with abnormal CT imaging are listed in Table 10. GCS is strongly linked to imaging abnormalities with abnormal CT scans in about 5% of patients with a GCS of 15 versus 30% when the GCS is 13 [10].

Patients with none of the factors in Table 10 or a normal CT with a GCS of 15 can usually be discharged for home observation; while patients with an abnormal CT or a GCS <15 generally need to be admitted [10].

Table 10 Factors associated with imaging abnormalities after a mild head injury. (Based on Ibañez 2004, Saboori 2007.)

- Age >60 years

- Coagulopathy

- Extracranial lesions

- Focal neurological deficit

- GCS <15

- Headache

- Hydrocephalus with shunt insertion

- Loss of consciousness

- Post-trauma amnesia

- Post-trauma seizure

- Skull fracture

- Vomiting

Testing women during pregnancy or while breastfeeding

The same principles concerning evaluation of headache in non-pregnant patients apply to women during pregnancy and lactation. Evaluations should not be delayed until after delivery or discontinuation of nursing and should include a detailed history, physical examination, and any necessary laboratory testing. The differential diagnosis should include consideration for eclampsia, thrombotic disease, benign intracranial hypertension (formerly called pseudotumor cerebri), or growth of pituitary adenomas or meningiomas.

Radiographic studies

Radiographic imaging of the cervical spine is typically delayed until after delivery, unless treatment will be altered based on results during pregnancy. Patients requiring x-rays should be provided with a pelvic shield to reduce fetal radiation exposure.

Neuroimaging studies should be considered when the patient's history or examination suggests neurological conditions for which an imaging study will potentially alter treatment during pregnancy. Similar to non-pregnant patients, MRI is preferred for pregnant and nursing patients being evaluated for headache. The American College of Radiology recommends MRI during pregnancy to avoid exposure to ionizing radiation when imaging studies are needed and the results of testing may change patient care [11]. MRI exposure during pregnancy is generally considered to be safe [12], with no negative sequelae identified during evaluation of three-year-olds exposed to MRI *in utero* [13] or the offspring of female MRI technicians [14].

CT imaging may be necessary in some women with abnormal neurological examinations or headaches suggesting intracranial hemorrhage. Fetal effects depend on both the timing and dosage of radiation exposure [15]. In general, fetal radiation exposure from a maternal head CT is extremely low (<0.005mGy), well below levels that have been linked to fetal effects [16-18]. Fetal exposure to ionizing radiation from a maternal head CT is generally considered to be substantially less risky for the fetus than not identifying and treating potentially serious neurological conditions in the mother [19].

The 11th European Symposium on Urogenital Radiology conducted an extensive literature review of the use of iodinated and gadolinium contrast during pregnancy and lactation, with a recommendation to use contrast agents when they are deemed necessary during pregnancy and nursing [20].

Iodinated contrast may be used during pregnancy if necessary information will be gathered from the testing. Exposure to maternal iodinated contrast agents can depress fetal and neonatal thyroid function; therefore, exposed newborns should be screened for thyroid function. There are no known fetal effects from intra-uterine gadolinium exposure. Only small amounts of iodinated or gadolinium contrast agents are expected in breast milk; therefore, temporary cessation of breastfeeding is not recommended when either contrast agent is used in lactating women.

Spinal fluid assessment

Spinal fluid examinations can be safely performed and easily interpreted in pregnancy, with opening pressure, cell count, and protein levels similar between non-pregnant and pregnant women [21]. Spinal fluid results are unaffected by active labor, length of gestation, and type of delivery (vaginal versus Cesarean section). Therefore, abnormal values obtained during pregnancy should not be attributed to the pregnancy itself, but must be further evaluated as in the non-pregnant patient.

Conclusions

All patients reporting a complaint of headache will require a detailed history and physical examination. Medical, neurological, and musculoskeletal evaluations are necessary to complete the headache work-up. A minority of patients will require specialized testing, such as radiographic studies, blood tests, or a spinal fluid examination. Identification of red flags, such as trauma, new onset headache, change in previous headache pattern, age >50 years old, and additional medical or neurological symptoms or signs, can help select patients requiring supplemental testing.

Key Summary

◆ History is the key to diagnostic assessment.

◆ Daily diaries can provide valuable information to clarify headache patterns and medication use.

◆ Patients with examinations suggesting possible secondary headaches may require supplemental evaluation with blood tests, radiographic studies, and/or spinal fluid analysis.

◆ Neuroimaging can be used in patients with likely secondary headaches during pregnancy and lactation.

◆ Patients with a mild head injury often develop headache and will need a detailed assessment of injury severity and impact.

References

1. Sandrini G, Friberg L, Jänig W, *et al.* Neurophysiological tests and neuroimaging procedures in non-acute headache: guidelines and recommendations. *Eur J Neurol* 2004; 11: 217-224.
2. Gore DR. Roentgenographic findings in the cervical spine in asymptomatic persons. A ten-year follow-up. *Spine* 2001; 26: 2463-2466.
3. Gore DR, Sepic SB, Gardner GM. Roentgenographic findings of the cervical spine in asymptomatic people. *Spine* 1986; 11(6): 521-524.
4. Marcus DA. Central nervous system abnormalities in migraine. *Expert Opin Pharmacother* 2003; 4: 1709-1715.
5. Ernst CW, Stadnik TW, Peeters E, Breucq C, Osteaux MJ. Prevalence of annular tears and disc herniations on MR images of the cervical spine in symptom-free volunteers. *Eur J Radiol* 2005; 55: 409-414.
6. Roos KL. Lumbar puncture. *Semin Neurol* 2003; 23: 105-114.
7. Meares S, Shores EA, Taylor AJ, *et al.* Mild traumatic brain injury does not predict acute postconcussion syndrome. *J Neurol Neurosurg Psychiatry* 2008; 79: 300-306.

8. Ibañez J, Arikan F, Pedraza S, *et al.* Reliability of clinical guidelines in the detection of patients at risk following mild head injury: results of a prospective study. *J Neurosurg* 2004; 100: 825-834.

9. Saboori M, Ahmadi J, Farajzadegan Z. Indications for brain CT scan in patients with minor head injury. *Clin Neurol Neurosurg* 2007; 109: 399-405.

10. Holm L, Cassidy JD, Carroll LJ, Borg J. Summary of the WHO Collaborating Centre for Neurotrauma Task Force on Mild Traumatic Brain Injury. *J Rehabil Med* 2005; 27:137-141.

11. ACR standards: MRI safety and sedation. Available at http://acr.org. Accessed March 2008.

12. Levine D, Barnes PD, Edleman RR. Obstetric MR imaging. *Radiology* 1999; 211: 609-17.

13. Baker P, Johnson I, Harvey P, Mansfield P. A three-year follow-up of children imaged *in utero* using echo-planar magnetic resonance. *Am J Obstet Gynecol* 1994; 170: 32-3.

14. Kanal E, Gillen J, Evans J, Savitz D, Shellock F. Survey of reproductive health among female MR workers. *Radiology* 1993; 187: 395-399.

15. Patel SJ, Reede DL, Katz DS, Subramaniam R, Amorosa JK. Imaging the pregnant patient for nonobstetric conditions: algorithms and radiation dose considerations. *Radiography* 2007; 27: 1705-1722.

16. American College of Obstetricians and Gynaecologists Committee Opinion. Guidelines for diagnostic imaging during pregnancy. *Obstet Gynecol* 2004; 104: 647-651.

17. Lowe SA. Diagnostic radiography in pregnancy: risks and reality. *Aust NZ J Obstet Gynaecol* 2004; 44: 191-196.

18. McCollough CH, Schueler BA, Atwell TD, *et al.* Radiation exposure and pregnancy: when should we be concerned? *Radiographics* 2007; 27: 909-918;

19. Dineen R, Banks A, Lenthall R. Imaging of acute neurological conditions in pregnancy and the puerperium. *Clin Radiol* 2005; 60: 1156-1170.

20. Webb JW, Thomsen HS, Morcos SK. The use of iodinated and gadolinium contrast media during pregnancy and lactation. *Eur Radiol* 2005; 15: 1234-1240.

21. Davis LE. Normal laboratory values of CSF during pregnancy. *Arch Neurol* 1979; 36: 443.

Chapter 3
Distinguishing primary from secondary headaches

Introduction

Most outpatient headaches evaluated in primary care are diagnosed as primary headaches [1]. Similarly, a recent study cataloguing headache diagnoses among outpatients referred to a tertiary headache center identified a minority of patients with secondary headaches (Table 1) [2]. Although headaches seen in the outpatient clinic are usually caused by primary headaches, especially migraine, correctly identifying secondary causes of headaches is the essential role of the headache evaluation. Patients without an identified secondary cause for headache may be categorized as having a primary headache disorder.

Distinguishing primary from secondary headaches

As described in Chapter 2, red flags suggesting a greater likelihood of a headache being caused by a secondary condition can be identified through a detailed history and physical examination (Table 2). In order to rule out possible secondary headaches, patients should be:

◆ queried about their current headaches and health problems;
◆ questioned about their previous headaches and medical conditions;
◆ asked to provide a complete review of systems.

Table 1 Diagnosis of tertiary care headache outpatients. (Based on Felício 2006.)

Headache category	Specific diagnosis	Percentage
Primary headaches		
	All primary diagnoses	83.8
	Migraine	52.3
	Tension-type	24.0
	Cluster	3.6
	Other	3.9
Secondary headaches		
	All secondary diagnoses	16.2
	Post-trauma	1.1
	Vascular disorder	0.3
	Non-vascular intracranial disorder	0.3
	Substance or its withdrawal	0.9
	Infection	0.4
	Homeostasis disorder	1.1
	Disorder of cranium, sinuses, teeth, or other cranial or facial structures	3.0
	Psychiatric disorder	0.3
	Neuralgia	2.8
	Other	6.1

Table 2 Features suggesting secondary headache.

- Patient ≥50 years old

- Significant change in headache quality or pattern for <2 years

- Pain in the posterior head or neck

- Additional medical symptoms

- Additional neurological symptoms

- Abnormal physical or neurological findings

General medical, neurological, and musculoskeletal examinations can help clarify a relationship between reported conditions or symptoms and the complaint of headache. For example, patients with arthritis who experience a restricted cervical spine range of motion and/or experience headache pain when changing neck posture are more likely to have an arthritic cause for headache than an arthritic patient with full cervical range of motion and no tenderness or pain reproduction with joint movement.

Headache conditions may be categorized as likely secondary or primary diagnoses, using information gleaned from the headache history questionnaire and physical examination (described in Chapter 2). Patient information can be applied to a diagnostic algorithm to quickly determine probable diagnoses (Figure 1).

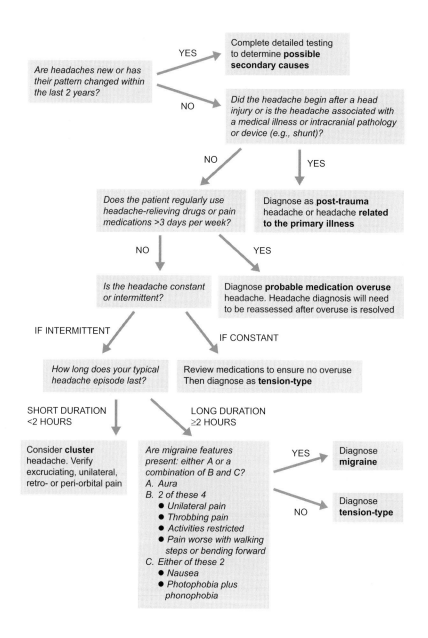

Figure 1 Diagnostic algorithm.

Secondary headaches

At the initial headache evaluation, most patients and their healthcare providers are primarily concerned with recognizing and correcting secondary causes of headache. Headache may be caused by a variety of medical conditions. While chronic headache is less likely to be caused by a secondary headache diagnosis, acute headache is also commonly caused by a primary headache disorder. Interestingly, migraine is the most common individual headache diagnosis seen in outpatients evaluated for acute headache. A survey of 561 patients seen in two primary care practices for a main complaint of acute headache reported a primary headache disorder for 56% of patients, with migraine the most common individual primary headache condition (81% of primary headaches and 45% of headaches overall) [3]. Secondary headaches were most commonly related to fever, hypertension, and sinusitis (Table 3).

Table 3 Secondary causes of acute outpatient headache. (Based on Bigal 2000.)

Secondary headache diagnosis	Percentage
All	44
Fever	16
Hypertensive peak	11
Sinusitis	8
Substance abuse	5
Post-trauma	2
Cervical disease	1
Expansive intracranial process	1
Intracranial infection (e.g., meningitis or brain abscess)	1
Dental fracture	<1
Post-dialysis	<1

Patients with features suggesting possible secondary headaches may need additional diagnostic testing targeted to specific disease states (as detailed in Chapter 2). Patients initially identified with a primary headache disorder may need to be reassessed for a possible secondary headache disorder if they:

◆ develop a new headache;
◆ experience a change in headache pattern;
◆ develop symptoms or signs of medical or neurological conditions;
◆ fail to improve with standard therapies designed for their primary headache disorder.

After reviewing the headache diary (provided in Chapter 2), important features that were not uncovered during the office visit may be identified, resulting in modification of the headache diagnosis.

Primary headaches

Primary headaches are distinguished by characteristic pain patterns, non-progressive character, and the absence of additional signs and symptoms [4]. Primary headaches are diagnosed by identifying characteristic patterns of headache symptoms.

Adult primary headaches

Primary headaches are distinguished by patterns of symptoms, including pain location, pain duration, and the behavioral response to headache (Table 4). Remember, patients with chronic headache who regularly use prescription or over-the-counter headache-relieving medication >3 days per week typically develop medication overuse headache. These patients should initially be diagnosed with medication overuse headache, with the diagnosis reassessed after the overuse medication has been discontinued for a couple of months, during which time the headache pattern will likely change.

Table 4 Distinguishing characteristics of adult primary headaches.

	Location	Typical duration (hours)	Preferred behaviors during headache
Migraine	Unilateral (affected side should vary at least occasionally)	8-24	Reduced productivity, lies down, seeks dark and quiet retreat
Tension-type	Bilateral	8-24 or constant	No interference with activities
Medication overuse	Bilateral	Constant with fluctuating severity	No interference with activities
Cluster	Unilateral eye (affected side will never vary)	½ - 1½	Avoids lying down, paces, smokes, showers, hits head

Migraine

Migraine is typically experienced as a disabling, intermittent headache lasting about 8-12 hours. A migraine attack can be divided into four stages: prodrome, aura, symptomatic, and postdrome (Table 5). A presymptomatic stage prodrome was historically considered to be a warning that a migraine attack was likely to occur. Today, most headache experts believe the prodrome actually represents the initial stages of a migraine attack already in progress rather than a premonition to a future migraine. Prodromes are recognized by about one in every three migraineurs [5]. Prodromal symptoms (Table 6) precede the symptomatic stages of migraine by an average of nine hours. Patients with prodromes are more likely to report migraine triggers and headaches of longer duration. Because neurochemical changes of migraine have probably already been initiated during the prodrome, patients with a prodrome may find that treating the prodrome with headache-relieving therapies can effectively abort the migraine before painful and disabling symptoms occur.

Table 5 Stages of migraine attack.

Features	Migraine stages			
	Prodrome	**Aura**	**Symptomatic**	**Postdrome**
% affected	30	15-20	100	70
Timing	Up to 48 hours before symptomatic phase	Immediately before symptomatic phase	After prodrome and aura	After symptomatic phase resolution
Duration	Hours-2 days	5-60 minutes	8-24 hours	Hours-1 day
Symptoms	Fatigue Mood change* GI symptoms** Pain Vision problems Sensitivity to noise or lights Dizziness Difficulty concentrating Food cravings	Scotoma Teichopsia Unilateral numbness	Unilateral, throbbing, disabling head pain Sensitivity to noises, lights, and smells Desire to isolate Nausea/vomiting	'Hung-over' Fatigue Loss of appetite Difficulty concentrating Low-grade discomfort

* Mood change may include irritability, euphoria, or depression
** Gastrointestinal (GI) symptoms may include diarrhea, constipation, or loss of appetite

Table 6 Percentage of migraine patients endorsing common prodromal symptoms. (Based on Kelman 2004.)

- Fatigue - 26%

- Mood change - 23%

- Gastrointestinal symptoms - 22%

- Head pain - 6%

About 15-20% of migraineurs experience a migraine aura about 30-60 minutes before the painful part of the attack. Auras are characteristically visual changes, including scotoma (described as blind spots) and teichopsia (described as zigzag lines). Other neurological phenomena, especially sensory changes, may also occur during an aura.

During the symptomatic stage of migraine, patients characteristically report a unilateral headache, although bilateral or holocranial pain is not uncommon. Features of migraine attacks were recently catalogued in 1283 patients (Table 7) [6]. Migraine sufferers typically modify their activities to accommodate their attacks, often finding comfort in reducing activity level and exposure to stimuli (like lights, sounds, smells, and food). Nausea and vomiting may accompany migraine, but most attacks will occur with only mild nausea or food aversion. With severe attacks, the migraineur characteristically retreats to a dark, quiet room and puts a washcloth over the eyes and forehead.

Table 7 Characteristics of average acute migraine episode. (Based on Kelman 2006.)

Headache feature	Average finding
Usual time of day with headache onset	53% anytime 19% morning 14% afternoon 4% evening 9% night
Time to peak headache severity	3 hours
Headache duration	29 hours
Headache intensity (0=none, 10=severe)	7
Throbbing pain	90%
Headache recurrence after treatment	44%
Time to headache recurrence	10 hours

Allodynia is another important migraine symptom, occurring in two of three migraineurs [7]. Common symptoms suggesting allodynia are listed in Table 8 [8]. Migraineurs typically find that headache-relieving therapies are more effective when administered before symptoms of allodynia occur [9]. Therefore, asking patients to monitor for allodynia is important when recommending timing for administering headache therapies. (Treatment details are provided in Chapter 5.)

Table 8 Symptoms of migraine-related allodynia.

Increase in pain occurs with:

- Combing the hair or wearing a ponytail

- Wearing glasses, contact lenses, or earrings

- Wearing a neck tie or tight clothing

- Shaving or showering

- Resting the face or head on a pillow

- Exposure to heat or cold

Table 9 Percentage of migraine patients endorsing common postdromal symptoms. (Based on Kelman 2006.)

- Fatigue - 72%

- Residual head pain - 33%

- Cognitive difficulties - 12%

- Feeling 'hung over' - 11%

- Gastrointestinal disturbance - 8%

- Mood disturbance - 7%

- Weakness - 6%

- Dizziness - 6%

A postdrome affects almost 70% of migraine patients (Table 9) [10]. Average postdrome duration is 25 hours. Migraineurs reporting a postdrome are also more likely to report a lower frequency headache and more migraine triggers.

Diagnostic pitfalls

Migraine sufferers often incorrectly attribute their headaches to sinus disease. Evaluation of 100 consecutive patients with self-diagnosed 'sinus' headache determined that 85% had migraine, while only 3% had headache associated with rhinosinusitis [11]. Among patients with definite migraine, several headache features were reported that resulted in the false attribution of headache to the sinuses (Table 10). Furthermore, migraine headaches will often respond to treatment with antihistamines, enhancing the false perception that the headaches are caused by sinus pathology.

Table 10 'Sinus' symptoms occurring during headache attacks in patients with definite migraine. (Based on Eross 2007.)

- Pain over sinus(es) - 97%

- Nasal congestion - 56%

- Eyelid edema - 37%

- Rhinorrhea - 25%

- Conjunctival injection - 22%

- Lacrimation - 19%

- Ptosis - 3%

- 'Sinus' triggers
  - Weather changes - 83%
  - Seasonal variation - 73%
  - Exposure to allergens - 62%
  - Change in altitude - 38%

Migraines are also incorrectly diagnosed as cluster headache in some cases. Interestingly, cluster patients rarely report autonomic features occurring with their headaches, probably because the intensity of the pain is so severe. Conversely, migraineurs frequently over-emphasize the occurrence and severity of autonomic symptoms with their headaches. A community survey of 841 migraineurs revealed one or more unilateral autonomic symptoms regularly occurring with migraine attacks in one in four migraineurs (Table 11) [12]. Autonomic symptoms were less frequently endorsed in this study compared with those in the previously described self-diagnosed 'sinus' headache study [11] because this study required regular and unilateral occurrence of autonomic symptoms with headache attacks rather than any occurrence used in the 'sinus' study.

Table 11 Unilateral 'cluster' symptoms regularly occurring during headache in patients with definite migraine. (Based on Obermann 2007.)

- Any unilateral symptom - 27%

- Lacrimation - 11%

- Conjunctival injection - 7%

- Ptosis/miosis - 5%

- Nasal congestion/rhinorrhea - 5%

- Eyelid edema - 4%

Tension-type

A tension-type headache is a milder, usually bilateral headache that does not interfere with activities. Tension-type headaches, however, often last one or several days, with some patients reporting daily or nearly daily headache. Sensitivity to stimuli is also not characteristic of a tension-type headache. Because of the milder nature of a tension-type headache, this is an infrequently diagnosed headache in typical medical practices.

Cluster headache

Cluster headaches often occur in groups or clusters, with the patient usually headache-free except for one to two annual clusters of attacks each lasting about six weeks, typically occurring in the spring and fall. During a cluster period, episodes tend to occur about 90 minutes after falling asleep, when entering dream sleep. Patients wake with a severe orbital pain that drives them out of bed. During the episode, the cluster patient often paces, showers, and smokes. Many patients severely press their eye or hit their head against the wall or books. Fortunately, each episode is relatively brief, resolving after about 30-90 minutes. During a cluster period, daytime attacks may be precipitated by using nicotine or alcohol. Generally, patients experience about one to three severe pain episodes nightly during a cluster period, with a lower frequency during the beginning and end of the cluster.

Pediatric primary headaches

In children presenting with acute headache, infectious etiologies, such as viral illness and sinusitis, are common and should be considered [13]. Imaging studies of the head are best reserved for children who have experienced traumatic or progressive headache, have a history of neurological illness (e.g., hydrocephalus), or have an abnormal neurological examination [14]. As in adult populations, children who experience a significant change in chronic headache pattern, chronic progressive headaches, or failure to respond to standard therapy may also need additional medical and neurological evaluations, including an imaging study.

Migraine

Children with migraine are less likely to endorse adult hallmark characteristics of migraine (Table 12) [15]. Although both children and adults report disabling headaches, pediatric migraine is more likely to:

◆ be bilateral;
◆ have a shorter duration (often <2 hours);
◆ lack reports of photophobia and phonophobia.

Pediatric migraine is typically diffuse and frontotemporal in location. Occipital headaches are unusual in children and should warrant consideration of a more extensive work-up.

Table 12 Diagnostic distinctions between pediatric and adult migraine. (Based on The International Classification of Headache Disorders, 2nd edition, 2004.)

	Adult	Pediatric
Location	Unilateral	Usually bilateral. Occipital migraine is rare and warrants additional evaluation
Duration	4-72 hours	1-72 hours
Associated symptoms	Photophobia and phonophobia are usually present	Children rarely verbalize sensitivity to noise and lights; photo- and phonophobia may be inferred from behavior (e.g. retreating to dark, quiet room; turning off television or computer)

A survey of high school students identified migraine in one in five students [16]. Among those qualifying for a diagnosis of migraine, characteristic adult features, especially unilateral pain, associated nausea, and throbbing pain were only endorsed by a minority of students (Figure 2). A survey of pediatric migraine patients similarly reported lack of adult migraine features, especially in younger patients [17]. Younger children were most likely to lack adult migraine characteristics. In comparison with adolescents, younger children reported a shorter average duration of headache (9 vs. 15 hours), a greater likelihood of being unable to describe headache pain ("It's just there:" 19% vs. 8%), and frontal pain location (56% vs. 46%). Other comparisons are shown in Table 13. In another survey of migraine patients (ages 9-16 years old), diaries showed that one in five had migraine episodes lasting less than one hour [18].

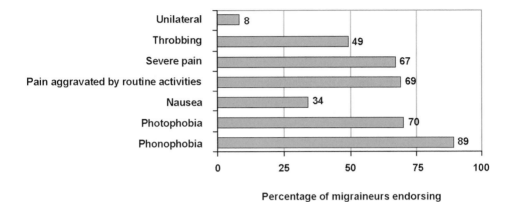

Figure 2 Prevalence of migrainous features in high school students with migraine. (Based on Unalp 2007.)

Table 13 Migrainous features in younger and older pediatric migraine patients. (Based on Hershey 2005.)

Migraine features	Migraine patients %	
	≤12 years old	>12 years old
Unilateral pain	28	27
Throbbing pain	62	75
Moderate-severe pain	95	94
Photophobia	75	84
Phonophobia	72	71
Combined photo- and phonophobia	63	66
Nausea	69	61

Name: _____

Date: _____/_____/_____

Time of day	Severity				Medications
	None	Mild	Moderate	Severe	
Morning					
Noon					
Evening					
Bedtime					

Check off any of the following that describe this headache:

☐ The pain affected one side of the head

☐ The pain felt like your heart beating in your head

☐ You had to stop what you were doing because of the headache

☐ You felt more comfortable when you turned off lights

☐ You felt more comfortable when it was quiet

☐ You felt sick to your stomach or threw up

When you got your headache:

Did your vision change?   YES   NO

Did you get dizzy?   YES   NO

Did you want to go to bed?   YES   NO

Draw a picture of your headache:

Figure 3 Pediatric headache diary.

Pediatric headache diagnostic tools

Because children often fail to verbally express migrainous features, pediatric headache diaries may help reveal migraine features that are not identified during clinical interview (Figure 3). Migraine features that were initially unrecognized on interview but later identified after diary review in one study included aura (46%), vomiting (50%), nausea (31%), unilateral location (38%), throbbing quality (29%), photophobia (11%), and phonophobia (11%) [19]. Thus, the use of diaries that instruct children to focus on certain symptoms improves the description of those headaches as migraine. Headache diaries are important not only to establish a headache diagnosis, but also to identify headache frequency in children. A comparison of impressions identified at a medical interview versus review of a headache diary showed identification of frequent (weekly) headache in only 18% during interviews compared with 48% when diaries were reviewed [20].

Another useful tool for uncovering pediatric migraine symptoms is to ask children to draw a picture of their headaches. When asked to draw what their headache feels like, children consistently produce features that can help distinguish migraine from a tension-type headache (Table 14) [21]. In one study, diagnostic accuracy from children's headache drawings was compared with a standard clinical assessment [22]. Headache drawings effectively depicted migraine features, with a diagnostic sensitivity of 93%, specificity of 83%, and positive predictive value of 87%. A later study further showed that comparing pre- with post-treatment headache drawings by children provides a good measure of treatment efficacy [23].

Table 14 Typical features seen on pediatric headache patient drawings. (Based on Wojaczynska-Stanek 2008.)

Migraine	Tension-type
Sharp elements - 55%	Compression elements - 55%
• Lightning	• Net
• Arrows pointing AWAY from head	• Something on head
• Needles	• Cap
• Nails	• Band
• Hammers	• Tongs
Part of the head - 28%	• Hands squeezing
• Half a head	Pressing elements - 17%
• Cracked head	• Weight on head
Noise - 10%	• Hammer
Electric current - 8%	Sharp elements - 11%
	• Arrows pointing TOWARD head

Pediatric migraine variants

A migraine equivalent syndrome occurs in one in ten patients seeing a pediatric neurologist for migraine [24]. The most common variant syndrome is benign paroxysmal vertigo. Cyclic vomiting, abdominal migraine, benign paroxysmal torticollis, and acute confusional state are other common syndromes.

Migraine variant syndromes may be considered after the exclusion of secondary causes of pediatric symptoms. A hallmark of each disorder is normalcy between symptomatic episodes. Patients with migraine variants should have normal neurological examinations, radiographic studies, and electroencephalography. Electroencephalography can be helpful in differentiating seizure from migraine in children with paroxysmal disorders. Migraine equivalents should be considered in pediatric patients with recurrent disorders, who have completed negative medical evaluations, particularly when a strong family history of migraine is present.

Benign paroxysmal vertigo

Benign paroxysmal vertigo typically occurs in young children, with episodes of short-lasting, severe balance disturbance initially occurring more frequently, with frequency diminishing with increasing age (Table 15) [25]. Symptoms often resolve by age 5.

Table 15 Benign paroxysmal vertigo. (Based on Drigo 2001.)

- Onset between 2-4 years old for 74% cases
  - Average age at onset=2.5 years old

- Often resolves by age 5

- Episodes of marked unsteadiness lasting several seconds to minutes
  - <5 minutes for 68% of cases

- Frequency 1-2 episodes per month in 68% of cases

- Asymptomatic between attacks

- Often associated with nystagmus and vomiting

- Family history of migraine in 53%

- These children usually develop migraine when older

Cyclic vomiting

Cyclic vomiting affects infants and young children and may be considered in otherwise healthy children with unexplained nausea and vomiting in whom symptoms are sudden in onset, self-limited with no symptoms between attacks, and accompanied by pallor and lethargy (Table 16) [26]. As described by the term cyclic, vomiting episodes tend to recur one or more times per month.

Table 16 Cyclic vomiting syndrome. (Based on Al-Twaijri 2002 and Dignan 2001.)

- Infants and children
  - Average onset at 3.6 years old

- Repeated bouts of explosive vomiting lasting hours to several days

- Asymptomatic between spells

- Usually associated with pallor and lethargy

- One in three also report headache, photophobia, or phonophobia with attacks

- One in three continue to have episodes into teens

- Family history of migraine in 65%

- Migraine develops in 46%

Abdominal migraine

Abdominal migraine is experienced as episodic bouts of moderate to severe midline abdominal pain, often associated with nausea, vomiting, and pallor (Table 17). Gastrointestinal testing is normal. Abdominal migraine typically begins in older children than cyclic vomiting.

Table 17 Abdominal migraine. (Based on Al-Twaijri 2002.)

- Children
  - Average onset at 7.6 years old

- Episodic, midabdominal pain lasts hours to several days

- Asymptomatic between attacks

- Usually associated with pallor

- Family history of migraine in 65%

- These children usually develop migraine when older

Benign paroxysmal torticollis

Benign paroxysmal torticollis typically affects infants and very young children, with frequency of episodes decreasing with age [27, 28]. Episodes of head tilt, vomiting, and ataxia may last hours to days (Table 18). Benign paroxysmal torticollis generally resolves during the preschool years. Radiographic studies of the head and neck should be routinely performed in children with paroxysmal torticollis.

Table 18 Benign paroxysmal torticollis. (Based on Al-Twaijri 2002.)

- Infants and very young children
  - Average age at onset = 1.2 years

- Episodes of head tilt, vomiting, and ataxia lasting hours to days

- Asymptomatic between attacks

- Family history of migraine in 73%

Acute confusional state

Acute confusional state is a rare migraine equivalent and must be differentiated from other causes of acute delirium [29, 30]. Episodes typically last minutes to hours (Table 19). As with other migraine equivalents, acute confusional state tends to resolve in early childhood and be replaced with migraine headache episodes [31].

Table 19 Acute confusional state. (Based on Al-Twaijri 2002.)

- Older children
  - Average onset at 10.9 years old

- Sudden onset of agitation, language dysfunction, memory disturbance, and confusion

- Episodes typically last minutes to hours - often resolve with sleep

- Asymptomatic between attacks - child often amnestic for episode

- Family history of migraine in 100%

- May occur after minor head injury

Conclusions

The majority of patients requesting evaluation for non-traumatic headache will have a primary headache condition. Identification of specific headache patterns can help distinguish among the common primary headache disorders. Pediatric migraine differs substantially from adult migraine. Migraine in children tends to be bilateral, of short duration, and less frequently associated with characteristic adult migraine features, such as throbbing pain and sensitivity to external stimulation. The diagnosis of childhood migraine can be facilitated by using a symptom checklist with the daily diary and asking children to draw pictures of their headache symptoms.

Key Summary

◆ Most acute and chronic headaches seen in outpatient practices are caused by primary headaches, especially migraine.

◆ Headaches that are new onset, changed in pattern, associated with additional symptoms or signs, or fail to respond to standard headache-relieving therapies should be evaluated as possible secondary headaches.

◆ Adult migraines can be divided into four stages: prodrome, aura, symptomatic, and postdrome.

◆ Migraines are often misdiagnosed as sinus or cluster headaches.

◆ Unlike adult migraines, pediatric migraines are often bilateral, shorter in duration, and lacking reports of throbbing pain, photophobia, or phonophobia.

◆ Diaries targeting migraine symptoms and headache drawings can help identify pediatric migraine patterns.

◆ Migraine variants cause episodic, non-painful disorders in infants and children.

References

1. Tepper SJ, Dahlöf CH, Dowson A, *et al.* Prevalence and diagnosis of migraine in patients consulting their physician with a complaint of headache: data from the Landmark study. *Headache* 2004; 44: 856-864.
2. Felício AC, Bischuette DB, dos Santos WC, *et al.* Epidemiology of primary and secondary headaches in a Brazilian tertiary-care center. *Arq Neuropsiquiatr* 2006; 64: 41-44.
3. Bigal ME, Bordini CA, Speciali JG. Etiology and distribution of headaches in two Brazilian primary care units. *Headache* 2000; 40: 241-247.
4. Ramirez-Lassepas M, Espinosa CE, Cicero JJ, *et al.* Predictors of intracranial pathological findings in patients who seek emergency care because of headache. *Arch Neurol* 1997; 54: 1506-1509.
5. Kelman L. The premonitory symptoms (prodrome): a tertiary care study of 893 migraineurs. *Headache* 2004; 44: 865-872.
6. Kelman L. Pain characteristics of the acute migraine attack. *Headache* 2006; 46: 942-953.
7. Lipton RB, Bigal ME, Ashina S, *et al.* Cutaneous allodynia in the migraine population. *Ann Neurol* 2008; 63: 148-158.
8. Jakubowski M, Silberstein S, Ashkenazi A, Burstein R. Can allodynic migraine patients be identified interictally using a questionnaire? *Neurology* 2005; 65: 1419-1422.
9. Burstein R, Collins B, Jakubowski M. Defeating migraine pain with triptans: a race against the development of cutaneous allodynia. *Ann Neurol* 2004; 55: 19-26.
10. Kelman L. The postdrome of the acute migraine attack. *Cephalalgia* 2006; 26: 214-220.
11. Eross E, Dodick D, Eross M. The Sinus, Allergy, Migraine Study. *Headache* 2007; 47(2): 213-224.
12. Obermann M, Yoon MS, Dommes P, *et al.* Prevalence of trigeminal autonomic symptoms in migraine: a population-based study. *Cephalalgia* 2007; 27(6): 504-509.
13. Burton LJ, Quinn B, Pratt-Cheney JL, Pourani M. Headache etiology in a pediatric emergency department. *Pediatr Emerg Care* 1997; 13: 1-4.
14. Kan L, Nagelberg J, Maytal J. Headaches in a pediatric emergency department: etiology, imaging, and treatment. *Headache* 2000; 40: 25-29.
15. Headache Classification Committee of the International Headache Society. The International Classification of Headache Disorders, 2nd edition. *Cephalalgia* 2004; 24(suppl1): 24-25.
16. Unalp A, Dirik E, Kurul S. Prevalence and clinical findings of migraine and tension-type headache in adolescents. *Ped Int* 2007; 49: 943-949.
17. Hershey AD, Winner P, Kabbouche MA, *et al.* Use of the ICHD-II criteria in the diagnosis of pediatric migraine. *Headache* 2005; 45: 1288-1297.
18. Van den Brink M, Badell-Hoekstra EG, Abu-Saad HH. The occurrence of recall bias in pediatric headache: a comparison of questionnaire and diary data. *Headache* 2001; 41: 11-20.
19. Metsähonkala L, Sillanpää M, Tuominen J. Headache diary in the diagnosis of childhood migraine. *Headache* 1997; 37: 240-244.

20. Laurell K, Larsson B, Eeg-Olofsson O. Headache in schoolchildren: agreement between different sources of information. *Cephalalgia* 2003; 23: 420-428.

21. Wojaczynska-Stanek K, Koprowski R, Wróbel Z, Gola M. Headache in children's drawings. *J Child Neurol* 2008; 23: 184-191.

22. Stafstrom CE, Rostasy K, Minster A. The usefulness of children's drawings in the diagnosis of headache. *Pediatrics* 2002; 109: 460-472.

23. Stafstrom CE, Goldenholz SR, Dulli DA. Serial headache drawings by children with migraine: correlation with clinical headache status. *J Child Neurol* 2005; 20: 809-813.

24. Al-Twaijri WA, Shevell MI. Pediatric migraine equivalents: occurrence and clinical features in practice. *Pediatr Neruol* 2002; 26: 365-368.

25. Drigo P, Carli G, Laverda AM. Benign paroxysmal vertigo of childhood. *Brain Dev* 2001; 23: 38-41.

26. Dignan F, Symon DK, ABuArafeh I, Russell G. The prognosis of cyclic vomiting syndrome. *Arch Dis Child* 2001; 84: 55-57.

27. Del Cuore F. Benign paroxysmal torticollis in childhood. *Pediatr Med Chi* 1997; 19: 69-70.

28. Balslev T, Falrup M, Ostergaard JR, Haslam RH. Benign paroxysmal torticollis. Recurrent involuntary twisting of the head in infants and young children. *Ugeskr Laeger* 1998; 160: 5365-5367.

29. Amit R. Acute confusional state in childhood. *Childs Nerv Syst* 1998; 4: 255-258.

30. D'Cruz OF, Walsh DJ. Acute confusional migraine: case series and review of literature. *Wis Med J* 1992; 91: 130-131.

31. Ehyai A, Fenichel GM. The natural history of acute confusional migraine. *Arch Neurol* 1978; 35: 368-369.

Chapter 4
Pathophysiology of chronic headaches

Introduction

Pain-sensitive structures in the head include the skin, bone, sinuses, blood vessels, and muscles. The brain parenchyma is insensate to pain, similar to other viscera. Secondary headaches generally occur because of traction, inflammation, bony abnormality, or increased intracranial pressure affecting pain-sensitive structures. Primary headaches are believed to occur due to activation of neural pain pathways within the brain. Imbalances in neurotransmitter levels or activity are postulated to result in most primary headaches. The best studied neurochemical abnormality in primary headache is an imbalance in serotonin.

Physiology of primary headaches

Migraine

Historically, migraine headache was considered to be caused by vascular dysfunction. Migraine is currently believed to represent a primarily neural disorder, with vascular changes occurring as a consequence of changes in neural activity. Migraine can be divided into three phases of pathogenesis [1]:

◆ brainstem neuronal hyperexcitability;
◆ cortical spreading depression with aura;
◆ trigeminal activation with complex migraine symptoms.

Brainstem hyperexcitability

Prior to developing a migraine aura or the symptomatic stage of migraine, migraineurs exhibit brainstem activation. Inherited abnormalities in calcium channel or other genes may contribute to this neuronal hyperexcitability. It has been postulated that pre-attack activation of brainstem structures may make migraineurs more susceptible to a variety of potential migraine trigger factors.

Cortical spreading depression

Cortical spreading depression was first described by Leão [2, 3]. Despite the name, cortical spreading depression first represents a slow progression across the cortex of short-lived neuronal excitation, followed by a more prolonged reduction in cortical activity. The rate of spread (about 2-6mm/minute) corresponds to the description of scotoma progression across the visual field during a migraine attack by Lashley [4]. Therefore, most experts believe that migraine aura occurs as a result of cortical spreading depression.

Mild cerebral ischemia follows cortical spreading depression. The neural nature of migraine pathogenesis is supported by the demonstration of cortical spreading depression progressing along non-vascular distributions.

Trigeminal activation

Trigeminal activation is the central feature of the neurovascular model of migraine proposed by Moskowitz [5]. During a migraine, nerve messengers signal the trigeminal system, a major pain relay station. Trigeminal signals reach a variety of structures, causing a complex assortment of migraine symptoms (Table 1 and Figure 1). Trigeminal activation may also cause increased sensitivity of the skin during migraine, causing allodynia.

Table 1 Consequences of trigeminal activation.

Structure activated	Symptom produced
Meningeal blood vessels	Increased blood flow and throbbing pain
Hypothalamus	Cravings
Cervical spine	Neck muscle tension and pain
Thalamus and cortex	Head pain

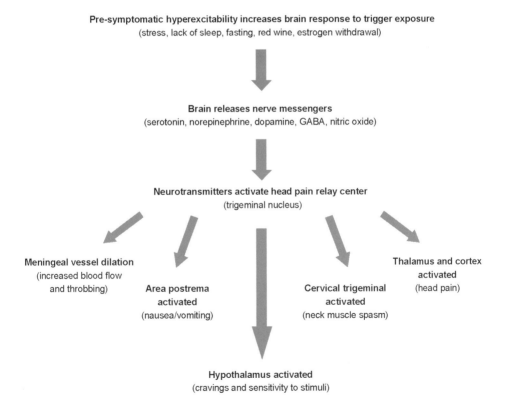

Figure 1 Model of migraine pathogenesis. (GABA=gamma-aminobutyric acid.)

Neurochemical dysfunction in migraine

A wide range of neurotransmitters are important in the pathogenesis of migraine (Table 2). Effective acute headache-relieving and prevention medications work by influencing target neurotransmitters, most commonly serotonin (Table 3). Early clinical trial data show similar good efficacy between a novel oral calcitonin gene-related peptide (CGRP) receptor antagonist [MK-0974] and rizatriptan [Maxalt], suggesting a future new class of effective oral, acute migraine treatment [6]. Because CGRP receptor antagonists lack direct vasoconstrictor properties, this class of medications may provide a useful alternative for patients unable to use triptans because of cardiovascular risk factors or those failing to achieve an adequate response from acute triptan therapy.

Table 2 Neurochemicals important for migraine.

- Serotonin (5HT)

- Gamma-aminobutyric acid (GABA)

- Calcitonin gene-related peptide (CGRP)

- Norepinephrine

- Dopamine

- Nitric oxide

- Estrogen

- Endorphins/enkephalins

Table 3 Migraine treatments and their neurochemical targets.

Treatment	Target
Acute headache-relieving drugs	
Analgesics	Serotonin, endorphins/enkephalins
Triptans	Serotonin
Anti-emetics	Dopamine
MK-0974 (in development)	Calcitonin gene-related peptide
Prevention therapies	
Antidepressants	Serotonin, norepinephrine
Anti-epileptics	Gamma-aminobutyric acid

Serotonin is the most thoroughly evaluated neurotransmitter for migraine. Many headache medications work by reducing serotonergic activity. Acute, headache-relieving therapies work by activating pre-synaptic, auto-regulatory, inhibitory $5HT_1$ receptors present on the dorsal raphe nucleus. Prevention therapies typically act as antagonists toward post-synpatic, excitatory $5HT_2$ receptors. Some antidepressants impair reuptake of serotonin after initial release, similarly reducing post-synaptic serotonin activation long-term. Some migraine drugs, like methysergide, act as both an agonist at the $5HT_1$ receptor and antagonist toward the $5HT_2$ receptor.

Another important vasodilator and neurotransmitter is nitric oxide. Nitric oxide also activates matrix metalloproteases (MMP), which influence brain development and the blood brain barrier (BBB). Cortical spreading depression at the onset of migraine results in up-regulation of MMP-9, causing breakdown of the BBB and vascular extravasation [7]. These effects may help explain how medications and neurotransmitters outside of the BBB can gain access to the brain during a migraine. Furthermore, changes in brain fluid status attributed to MMP may explain the occurrence of non-specific white matter changes seen on magnetic resonance imaging studies in about 30% of migraineurs.

Sex hormones, especially estrogen, also exert a strong influence on migraine. Sex hormones are classified as neurosteroids, to highlight their important role in neural function. Estrogen is an important pain modulator, directly affecting nociceptive transmission within the central nervous system. For example, intracellular estrogen receptors exist in the majority of enkephalin-producing neurons in the superficial laminae of both spinal and trigeminal dorsal horns [8]. Estrogen exposure to these neurons results in increased enkephalin production by 68% [9]. Estradiol also increases levels of a variety of additional pain-modulating neurotransmitters, including 5HT, GABA, and endorphin [10, 11].

Genetic factors

About half to two-thirds of people with migraine will have close relatives with migraine, especially maternal relatives. A study of over 8000 adult twin pairs showed that when one twin had migraine, an identical twin was over twice as likely to also have migraine compared with a non-identical twin [12]. This study showed that about half the risk for migraine could be attributed to genetic factors.

Specific genetic mutations have been most consistently identified in a rare type of autosomal dominant migraine with unilateral paralysis or weakness during migraine attacks, called familial hemiplegic migraine. Mutations at three specific genes have been linked to familial hemiplegic migraine:

◆ chromosome 19 - alpha 1A subunit P/Q neural calcium channel gene (CACNA1A);
◆ chromosome 1 - alpha 2 subunit Na/K ATPase gene (ATP1A2);
◆ chromosome 2q24 - neuronal voltage-gated sodium channel (SCN1A).

Consistent genetic abnormalities have not been widely identified in more typical migraine patients.

Iron homeostasis

Iron homeostasis in the peri-aqueductal grey matter may be an important marker of migraine activity. Peri-aqueductal grey iron homeostasis was evaluated in patients with episodic migraine (N=17), migraine transformed into chronic daily headache (N=17), and no headaches (N=17) [13]. Magnetic resonance imaging transverse relaxation values showed increased R2' values in migraineurs, denoting increased iron deposition with episodic migraine (6.11) and chronic daily headache (6.36) compared with controls (4.33). There were no differences between migraine with and without aura. Furthermore, migraine duration correlated linearly with iron deposition for both migraine groups. Although the significance of this finding is unclear, these data further support the biological basis of migraine and reinforce the need for effective intervention to hopefully reduce longstanding changes in cerebral markers.

Tension-type headache

The same pathophysiological changes seen in migraine may also be seen in patients with a tension-type headache [14]. In general, tension-type headache sufferers have the same qualitative changes as migraineurs, but the severity is less. For this reason, many headache specialists consider migraine and tension-type headache to be part of a continuum, with more severe pathology resulting in the more disabling symptoms of migraine and milder changes resulting in non-disabling tension-type headaches. Pathophysiological similarities also predict a similar ability of the same medication and non-medication treatments to generally work well for both migraine and tension-type headaches. For example, migraine-specific headache relieving triptans (including sumatriptan and rizatriptan) have also been shown to effectively treat non-migraine, tension-type headaches [15, 16].

Medication overuse headache

The pain-relieving effects of aspirin and acetaminophen may be at least partially explained by the effect of reducing cortical $5HT_2$ receptors [17, 18]. While intermittent analgesic use can effectively relieve headache pain, chronic, daily use results in an up-regulation of postsynaptic $5HT_2$ serotonin receptors [19]. This up-regulation increases firing of these pain-provoking receptors and may explain increased headache activity with prolonged and excessive use of analgesics or other serotonin-active medications such as the triptans. Serotonin receptor activation returns to normal levels slowly after medication withdrawal, typically requiring about three months for full correction. In support of this model, patients with medication overuse headache often require several months for headaches to improve to pre-medication overuse levels.

Post-trauma headache

A post-trauma headache occurs as a result of microscopic shearing forces that alter brainstem activity as the cortex moves above the relatively immobile brainstem at the time of impact. The dorsal midbrain is typically affected with head injury [20]. Researchers postulate that those same areas experiencing dysfunction in migraine may be damaged by axonal shearing, resulting in increased headache susceptibility after head trauma. Mild head injury with concussion produces alterations in serotonin and other brain chemicals, similar to changes seen in spontaneously-occurring migraine [21].

Cluster headache

The pathophysiology of cluster headaches is poorly understood, likely due to the relatively low prevalence of this disorder. Cluster headaches are similarly linked to trigeminal activation, although functional neuroimaging studies suggest a more pronounced role for the posterior hypothalamus grey matter in cluster headache, which may explain their circadian characteristics [22].

Conclusions

The exact pathophysiology of primary headaches is unknown, although changes in brain excitation and neurotransmitter activity seem to be important factors. Effective therapies targeting specific neurochemicals, such as serotonin and calcitonin gene-related peptide, further support the important role of neurotransmitters in primary headaches. Most studies describing pathogenesis of headache have utilized patients with migraine headache, with less data available for other primary headache disorders.

Key Summary

◆ Migraine results from brainstem excitation, cortical spreading depression, and trigeminal activation.

◆ Important changes in neurotransmitters, including serotonin, calcitonin gene-related peptide, and gamma-aminobutryic acid, have been targeted for the development of effective migraine therapies.

◆ Tension-type headaches appear to share pathological features with migraine.

◆ Medication overuse headaches may result from up-regulation of serotonin receptors in patients chronically exposed to analgesics or triptans.

◆ Patients with a cluster headache show abnormalities in the hypothalamus that may help explain the circadian patterns of this headache disorder.

References

1.	Arulmai U, Gupta S, Maassen VanDenBrink A, *et al*. Experimental migraine models and their relevance in migraine therapy. *Cephalalgia* 2006; 26: 642-659.
2.	Leão AP. Spreading depression of activity in the cerebral cortex. *J Neurophysiol* 1944; 7: 359-390.
3.	Teive HA, Kowacs PA, Marahão Filho P, Piovesan EJ, Werneck LC. Leão's cortical spreading depression: from experimental 'artifact' to physiological principle. *Neurology* 2005; 65: 1455-1459.
4.	Lashley KS. Patterns of cerebral integration indicated by the scotomas of migraine. *Arch Neurol Psychiatry* 1941; 46: 331-339.
5.	Moskowitz MA. The neurobiology of vascular head pain. *Ann Neurol* 1984; 16: 157-168.
6.	Ho TW, Mannix LK, Fan X, *et al*. Randomized controlled trial of an oral CGRP receptor antagonist, MK-0974, in acute treatment of migraine. *Neurology*, in press.

7. Gursoy-Ozdemir Y, Qiu J, Matsuoka N, *et al.* Cortical spreading depression activates and upregulates MMP-9. *J Clin Investigation* 2004; 113(10): 1447-1455.

8. Amandusson A, Hermanson O, Blomqvist A. Colocalization of oestrogen receptor immunoreactivity and preproenkephalin mRNA expression to neurons in the superficial laminae of the spinal and medullary dorsal horn of rats. *Eur J Neurosci* 1996; 8: 2440-2445.

9. Amandusson A, Hallbeck M, Hallbeck AL, *et al.* Estrogen-induced alterations of spinal cord enkephalin gene expression. *Pain* 1999; 83: 243-248.

10. Joy KP, Tharakan B, Goos HJ. Distribution of gamma-aminobutyric acid in catfish (*Heteropneustes fossilis*) forebrain in relation to season, ovariectomy and E2 replacement, and effects of GABA administration on plasma gonadotropin-II level. *Comp Biochem Physiol A Mol Integr Physiol* 1999; 123: 369-376.

11. Lagrange AH, Ronnekleiv OK, Kelly MJ. The potency of mu-opioid hyperpolarization of hypothalamic arcuate neurons is rapidly attenuated by 17-beta-estradiol. *J Neurosci* 1994; 14: 6196-6204.

12. Honkasalo, M-L, Kaprio J, Winter T, *et al.* Migraine and concomitant symptoms among 8,167 adult twin pairs. *Headache* 1995; 35: 70-78.

13. Welch KM, Nagesh V, Aurora SK, Gelman N. Periaqueductal gray matter dysfunction in migraine: cause or the burden of illness? *Headache* 2001; 41(7): 629-637.

14. Marcus DA. Migraine and tension-type headaches: the questionable validity of current classification systems. *Clin J Pain* 1992; 8:2 8-36.

15. Lipton RB, Stewart WF, Cady R, *et al.* Sumatriptan for the range of headaches in migraine sufferers: results of the Spectrum Study. *Headache* 2000; 40: 783-791.

16. Allen C, Cady R, Lines C, McCarroll K. Effect of rizatriptan in the spectrum of headache. *Headache* 2001; 41: 607-608.

17. Pini LA, Vitale G, Sandrini M. Serotonin and opiate involvement in the antinociceptive effect of acetylsalicylic acid. *Pharmacology* 1997; 54: 84-91.

18. Pini LA, Sandrini M, Vitale G. The antinociceptive action of paracetamol is associated with changes in the serotonergic system in the rat brain. *Eur J Pharmacol* 1996; 308: 31-40.

19. Smith TR, Stoneman J. Medication overuse headache from antimigraine therapy. Clinical features, pathogenesis and management. *Drugs* 2004; 64: 2503-2514.

20. Hashimoto T, Nakamura N, Richard KE, Frowein RA. Primary brain stem lesions caused by closed head injuries. *Neurosurg Rev* 1993; 16: 291-298.

21. Packard RC, Ham LP. Pathogensis of posttraumatic headache and migraine: a common headache pathway? *Headache* 1997; 37(3): 142-152.

22. Goadsby PJ. Pathophysiology of cluster headache: a trigeminal autonomic cephalalgia. *Lancet Neurol* 2002; 1: 251-257.

Chapter 5
Treating headaches

Introduction

Headache medications can be divided into acute, headache-relieving drugs and prevention therapies. Acute medications are designed to treat a currently occurring headache episode. Acute medications need to be limited to a maximum of three days per week on a regular basis, or medication overuse headache can develop.

Prevention medications are designed to be used every day to help prevent future headaches from occurring. Most prevention medications take several weeks to months to achieve an effect, so taking an extra dosage during a headache episode will not improve that headache.

This chapter will describe acute and prevention treatments in typical adult headaches. Treating headaches in children and for women during different reproductive stages will be described in Chapter 8. The management of headaches in elderly patients will be covered in Chapter 10.

Acute treatment

Acute treatments should be used on a regular basis no more than three days per week to treat infrequent headache or more severe headache episodes in patients with frequent headache. Selection among available acute treatment options depends primarily on the severity of symptoms (Table 1). Anti-emetics provide a useful adjunctive therapy in patients with pronounced nausea associated with their intermittent, chronic headache episodes.

Table 1 Acute headache medications.

Mild, non-disabling headache
- Analgesics
    - Analgesic plus caffeine (most effective)
    - Aspirin
    - Non-steroidal anti-inflammatory drugs
    - Acetaminophen (less effective)

Moderate-severe or disabling headache
- Triptan (most effective)

- Ergotamine (less effective)

Associated nausea
- Anti-emetics (most effective)

- Metoclopramide (less effective)

Rescue therapy
- Non-opioid analgesics

- Short-acting opioids (less effective for headache than non-opioid analgesics)

Rescue therapy may be needed sporadically. Patients should understand that no individual acute therapy will be effective for every headache episode. Rescue therapy, therefore, has a role when patients are undergoing trials to identify effective acute therapy and for the occasional headache that fails to respond in patients who have otherwise achieved good headache control.

Analgesics

Aspirin and non-steroidal anti-inflammatory drugs are more effective than acetaminophen and opioids for reducing mild to moderate severity headaches. Adding 100mg of caffeine to acute analgesics improves the number of people getting headache relief by 1.5 times [1]. Therefore, first choice therapy for mild to moderate severity headaches is often an analgesic plus caffeine combination product or an analgesic taken with a caffeinated beverage.

The European Federation of Neurological Societies (EFNS) published evidence-based guidelines for migraine therapy in 2006 [2]. Recommended acute analgesics are listed in Table 2. Stronger evidence supports the use of first-line agents.

Table 2 EFNS acute analgesic migraine drug recommendations. (Based on Evers 2006.)

Acute analgesic therapy	Typical oral dose
First-line	
Acetylsalicylic acid/aspirin	1000mg
NSAIDs	Ibuprofen 200-800mg
	Naproxen 500-1000mg
	Diclofenac 50-100mg
Paracetamol/acetaminophen	1000mg
Analgesic plus caffeine	250mg aspirin
	200-250mg paracetamol
	50mg caffeine
Second-line	
Metamizol	1000mg
Phenazon	1000mg
Tolfenamic acid	200mg

Triptans

Triptans are particularly beneficial for patients with moderate to severe disabling attacks (Table 3). The choice of triptan is based on slight differences in time course of action and formulation preference (Figure 1). A comparison among different available triptans was performed using meta-analysis of data supplied by pharmaceutical companies that included double-blind, randomized, controlled clinical trials [3]. This analysis

Table 3 Triptans.

Triptan	Typical dosage	Attribute
Fastest acting Sumatriptan	6mg SQ 20mg NS	Relief may begin after 10-15 minutes Efficacy superior with SQ injection Efficacy similar for NS or PO, although relief is faster with NS
Zolmitriptan	5mg NS	Relief may begin after 10 minutes
Fast-acting Almotriptan	12.5mg PO	Fast-acting Good tolerability
Eletriptan	40-80mg PO	Fast-acting Excellent efficacy
Rizatriptan	10mg PO or orally disintegrating	Fast-acting Excellent efficacy
Sumatriptan	50-100mg PO	Fast-acting
Zolmitriptan	5mg PO or orally dissolving	Fast-acting
Slower acting Frovatriptan	2.5mg PO	Sustained effect, but efficacy relatively low Minimal number of side effects
Naratriptan	2.5mg PO	Sustained effect, but efficacy relatively low Minimal number of side effects

NS=nasal spray, PO=oral, SQ=subcutaneous

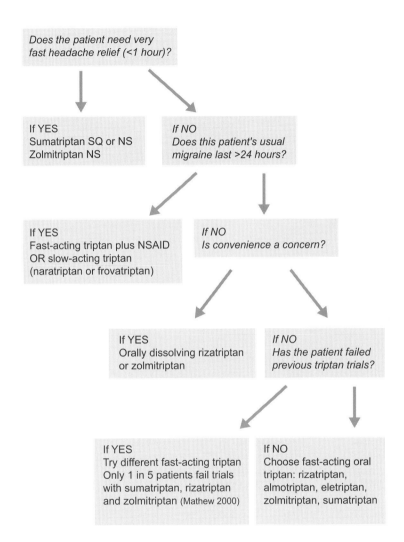

Figure 1 Selecting a triptan.

supported selecting rizatriptan, eletriptan, or almotriptan as first-line triptan therapy in patients needing a fast-acting oral triptan (Figure 2; Table 4) [3]. Frovatriptan and naratriptan are less effective than the oral, fast-acting triptans, although tolerability is superior.

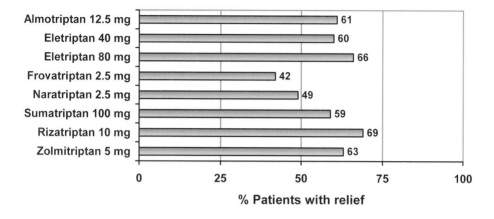

Figure 2 Efficacy comparison among triptans. Headache response was measured two hours after treatment. Relief denotes an improvement from moderate/severe pain to mild/no pain. (Based on Ferrari 2002.)

Table 4 Outcome comparison among triptans. Comparisons are made using sumatriptan 100mg response as the standard. (Based on Ferrari 2002.)

Triptan	2-hour relief	24-hour pain-free	Consistency	Tolerability
Almotriptan 12.5mg	Same	Better	Better	Much better
Eletriptan 40mg	Same-better	Same-better	Same	Same
Eletriptan 80mg	Better	Better	Same	Same
Frovatriptan 2.5mg	Worse	Worse	Worse	Much better
Naratriptan 2.5mg	Worse	Worse	Worse	Much better
Rizatriptan 10mg	Better	Better	Better	Same
Zolmitriptan 5mg	Same	Same	Same	Same

Most patients will respond to at least one of three triptan trials [4]. Migraine episodes with more severe symptoms are less likely to respond to treatment [5]; therefore, patients should treat several migraine episodes with a single triptan before abandoning that therapy as ineffective. Combining a triptan with an analgesic may increase the duration of headache relief [6]. For example, randomized, double-blind studies comparing sumatriptan 85mg plus naproxen 500mg versus either compound alone or placebo showed a superior (P<0.01) sustained pain-free response with the combination of sumatriptan and naproxen sodium (23-25% of patients) compared with sumatriptan monotherapy (14-16%), naproxen monotherapy (10%), or placebo (7-8%) [7].

Triptans should not be prescribed for patients with cardiovascular disease, ischemic bowel disease, uncontrolled hypertension, or severe liver disease. They should likewise not be used in patients treated with monoamine oxidase inhibitor antidepressants or ergotamines. Triptans are also restricted in patients with hemiplegic migraine or basilar migraine, a rare type of migraine associated with loss of consciousness and brainstem dysfunction.

Ergotamine

Ergotamine preparations also provide good efficacy for disabling headaches. Vasoconstrictive properties with ergotamines result in more significant side effects with ergotamines compared with triptans. Dihydroergotamine (DHE) is most effective and is typically administered as a 1mL dose intravenously, intramuscularly, or subcutaneously. Subcutaneous dosing can be self-administered by patients. DHE is also available as a 4mg/mL nasal spray and may be compounded as a sublingual preparation. The nasal spray is administered as one 0.5mg spray in each nostril, repeated once in 15 minutes.

DHE does not work as quickly as the fastest-acting triptans, but sustained response is better with DHE. Ergotamines should not be used in patients with cardiovascular or peripheral vascular disease or significant vascular risk factors. Patients with ischemic bowel disease or Raynaud's syndrome should also avoid ergotamines. Ergotamines should also not be used in patients taking triptans within the preceding 24 hours before DHE dosing. DHE is most commonly used in patients with recalcitrant, severe or prolonged migraines that have failed to respond to triptan therapy.

Anti-nausea drugs

Anti-emetics provide helpful adjunctive headache treatment for headache associated with nausea [8-10]. Anti-emetics are most helpful when used as supplemental therapy in combination with analgesic or other acute headache treatment. Monotherapy often results in only short-lived benefits. Several anti-emetics have demonstrated efficacy in acutely reducing headache symptoms in the literature (Table 5). The EFNS recommends metoclopramide and domperidone [2].

Table 5 Effective anti-emetics for acute episodes of chronic headache with nausea.

- Domperidone 20-30mg PO

- Prochlorperazine 2 mg PR

- Promethazine 12.5-25mg PR

- Metoclopramide 10mg PO or IM, 20 mg PR

- Ondansetron 4mg IV

IM=intramuscular, IV=intravenous, PO=oral, PR=rectal

Emerging therapy

Patients and their healthcare providers can be encouraged that, even if available treatments have not been helpful, chronic headache is an area of robust research and new pharmaceutical development. A wide variety of acute headache therapies targeting novel neural receptors are under various stages of development and testing. Several promising receptor targets and compounds are highlighted below.

Calcitonin gene-related peptide (CGRP) receptors may offer another important target for acute headache medications. Promising results have been published with an intravenous CGRP-antagonist [BIBN4096BS] and an oral preparation [MK-0974] [11]. Intravenous BIBN4096BS 2.5mg produced two-hour headache relief in 66% versus 27% with placebo. Early phase III clinical trial data show similar good efficacy between a novel oral CGRP receptor antagonist [MK-0974] and rizatriptan [12]. Two-hour pain relief similarly occurred in 68% treated with MK-0974 300mg versus 70% with rizatriptan 10mg. CGRP receptor antagonists lack direct vasoconstrictor properties and may offer an effective alternative for patients unable to use triptans because of cardiovascular risk factors or those failing to achieve an adequate response from acute triptan therapy.

Carbon dioxide may also have a role as an acute headache treatment. Experimental studies show the ability of CO_2 to inhibit sensory nerve activation and also inhibit CGRP secretion, suggesting possible mechanisms for relieving acute headaches [13]. Early phase II clinical trial data have shown the effectiveness of 100% CO_2 delivered intranasally at a flow rate of 10mL/second [14].

Vanilloid TRPV1 receptors are located on trigeminal and dorsal root ganglia and may be an additional receptor site target for pain and migraine therapies [15]. A preliminary clinical trial with TRPV1 receptor antagonist [SB705498] was terminated early, due to low efficacy; however, a variety of other compounds have been developed that may demonstrate better efficacy for migraine [15]. For example, another product [MK-2295] is currently under trials for relieving dental pain.

Nitric oxide is another chemical important in migraine pathogenesis. Nitric oxide synthetase inhibitor [GW274150] has established anti-inflammatory and analgesic properties [16]. Phase II clinical trials testing GW274150 for the acute treatment of migraine have been completed, although results have not yet been published.

Novel delivery systems may also improve efficacy of acute migraine treatments. Phase I clinical trials support the feasibility of administering sumatriptan using an iontophoretic transdermal patch, with fewer adverse events reported than with subcutaneous sumatriptan [17]. Future studies will evaluate clinical efficacy with iontophoretic patch delivery.

Monitoring acute treatment response

No acute headache medication will effectively treat every headache episode. For this reason, any new acute headache therapy should be tested on three separate headache episodes to accurately assess its efficacy (Table 6). Patients are often hesitant to use a medication the first

Table 6 Patient acute treatment satisfaction questionnaire.

Acute headache medication: _____	Headache #1 Date: / /		Headache #2 Date: / /		Headache #3 Date: / /	
How quickly did you get headache relief?						
Was relief *fast enough* for you?	YES	NO	YES	NO	YES	NO
Did your headache symptoms go away *completely*?	YES	NO	YES	NO	YES	NO
Did you have to *repeat your dose*?	YES	NO	YES	NO	YES	NO
Is the *formulation* you're using (tablet, dissolving tablet, nasal spray, or injection) convenient and effective for you?	YES	NO	YES	NO	YES	NO
Are you having *troublesome side effects* that make you hesitant to use your medication?	YES	NO	YES	NO	YES	NO
Overall, are you *satisfied* with this treatment?	YES	NO	YES	NO	YES	NO

time, waiting until their headache is very severe and, thereby, minimizing its effectiveness. Subsequent trials often reveal better efficacy, possibly due to treating the headache earlier and reduced patient anxiety about an unknown therapy.

Prevention

In general, headache prevention therapies are considered to be effective when they result in a 50% or better reduction in headache activity. Few drugs are FDA-approved as migraine preventive therapy (Table 7), with most preventives used based on clinical trials documenting benefit after drugs have been approved and available for treating other medical conditions, most commonly mood disorders, cardiovascular disease, and epilepsy. Non-approved drugs listed in the table have all shown efficacy in open-label or controlled clinical trials [18-24]. The EFNS has similarly recommended a variety of prevention therapies, divided into first-, second-, and third-line choices, based on available supportive evidence (Table 8) [2]. Prevention benefits from antidepressants are independent of effects on mood [25]. In all cases, therapies are generally best tolerated when initiated at low doses and slowly titrated as tolerated to achieve an effective maintenance dosage.

Long-acting opioids are generally not beneficial for chronic headaches. Even with the best management, long-acting opioids result in only modest benefit with a high risk of abuse. In a long-term study conducted using carefully selected chronic headache patients tightly monitored for compliance, long-acting opioids needed to be discontinued in three of every four patients [26].

Table 7 Headache prevention therapies.

Drug	Comorbidity treated	Typical maintenance dosage
FDA-approved drugs for migraine prevention		
Methysergide maleate	None	2mg three times daily Unavailable in the United States Previously used for recalcitrant migraine Associated with risks for pulmonary, endocardial, and retroperitoneal fibrosis Drug holiday required after 6 months of use
Propranolol	Hypertension Angina Hypertrophic subaortic stenosis Essential tremor	80-160mg long-acting form daily
Timolol	Hypertension	20mg daily
Divalproex sodium	Epilepsy Bipolar disorder with mania	125-250mg twice daily
Topiramate	Epilepsy Obesity	50-100mg twice daily
Non-approved prevention treatments		
Antidepressants	Depression Anxiety Sleep disturbance Fibromyalgia Neuropathic pain	Tricyclics are the most effective antidepressant class for headache prevention. e.g., amitriptyline or imipramine 25-100mg 2 hours before bed
Anti-epileptics	Neuropathic pain Anxiety Sleep disturbance	Gabapentin 100-400mg 2-3 times daily Levetiracetam 500mg twice daily Lamotrigine 50mg twice daily
Antihistamine	Infrequently used in adults due to sedation	Cinnarizine 25mg three times daily or 75mg at bedtime (unavailable in North America) Cyproheptadine 4mg 2-3 times daily
Calcium channel blockers	Hypertension Angina Arrhythmia	Less effective than beta-blockers. Flunarizine 5-10mg daily (not available in the United States, but more effective than verapamil) Verapamil 240-480mg long-acting form daily
Tizanidine	Myofascial pain Sleep disturbance	2-8mg two to three times daily

Table 8 EFNS prevention migraine drug recommendations. (Based on Evers 2006.)

Preventive therapy	Typical daily maintenance dosage
First-line	
Beta-blockers	Metoprolol 50-200mg
	Propranolol 40-240mg
Calcium channel blocker	Flunarizine 5-10mg
Neurostabilizing anti-epileptic	Topiramate 25-100mg
	Divalproex sodium 500-1800mg
Second-line	
Amitriptyline	50-150mg
Bisoprolol	5-10mg
Third-line	
Candesartan	16mg
Gabapentin	1200-1600mg
Lisinopril	20mg
Methysergide	4-12mg

Emerging therapy

Tonabersat is a new compound, currently in Phase II clinical trials as a migraine prevention therapy. Tonabersat is a gap junction blocker, inhibiting cortical spreading depression and its consequences in migraine pathogenesis. In a double-blind, placebo-controlled trial, patients with active migraine were treated with tonabersat initiated at 20mg daily for two weeks and increased to 40mg daily for an additional ten weeks [27]. Preliminary results were promising with a 50% or better reduction in headache realized for 62% treated with tonabersat versus 45% with placebo.

Occipital nerve stimulation has also been studied as a possible alternative preventive method for reducing trigeminal pain. In a small study, 15 patients with recalcitrant chronic headaches that included pain in the C2 distribution underwent temporary implantation of an occipital nerve stimulator [28]. Patient diagnoses included chronic migraine (N=8), chronic cluster (N=3), post-trauma headache (N=2), and hemicrania continua (N=2). Hemicrania continua is a rare type of long-lasting, unilateral headache that is described in Chapter 10. Electrode placement was bilateral in eight patients and unilateral in seven. Follow-up was performed after an average of 20 months. Mean change in headache pain was a 52% reduction, with a 50% or better reduction reported in nearly two of every three patients. Headache frequency was decreased by nearly one third. The most common adverse event was lead migration requiring surgical revision (N=8). Additional studies using larger sample sizes will be needed to confirm these preliminary positive results.

Monitoring treatment response

Benefit from preventive medication is not anticipated for several weeks to months. In many cases, benefits are only experienced after patients have been treated with a maintenance dosage for three to four weeks. Pre- and post-treatment diary comparisons are particularly beneficial for identifying an early response to prevention therapies. Initial benefit from preventive therapy is often experienced as a reduction in headache duration or overall severity rather than an increase in the number of totally headache-free days. For this reason, diaries requiring headache severity recording several times daily (see Chapter 2) are ideal for capturing early prevention benefits. Patients recording headache activity only once daily may miss important clues that therapy is beginning to be effective.

Patients using any prevention medication will need to be monitored for both efficacy and tolerability. Sedation and cognitive effects are common problematic side effects from headache prevention therapies. Furthermore, the Food and Drug Administration recently announced a warning about increased risk of suicide among patients using some anti-epileptic drugs, including gabapentin, pregabalin, topiramate, and valproate [29]. Change in mood can also occur in patients treated with beta-blocker antihypertensive medications.

Treating secondary headaches

Secondary headaches are primarily managed by treating the underlying condition responsible for the headache. During the course of treating that condition, persistent or residual headaches may be managed using acute or preventive medications listed above, as appropriate.

Medication overuse headache

Medication overuse headaches are primarily treated with medication withdrawal, followed by reassessment (Table 9). Additional headache acute or prevention therapies are typically ineffective while patients are overusing medications. Therefore, new therapies are generally not added until withdrawal is completed and headache reassessment has occurred.

Table 9 Treatment of probable medication overuse headache.

- Discontinue non-opioid analgesics and triptans

- Taper opioids, butalbital combinations, and ergotamines by one half to one pill per week

- Prescribe a low-dose non-ibuprofen non-steroidal anti-inflammatory drug or tramadol twice daily, with an additional dose permitted once daily for severe pain during first month after discontinuing analgesics or throughout period of taper

- Reassess headache pattern 1 month after discontinuing analgesics and triptans or completing drug taper

- Treat frequent headache with standard preventive headache therapy

- Limit acute medications to a maximum of 3 days per week for infrequent, severe headaches only

- Maintain headache diary to ensure no return of excessive acute care medication

---

Medication withdrawal can typically be successfully achieved in the outpatient setting. Formal detoxification programs are generally unnecessary. In one study, 120 otherwise healthy patients with medication overuse headache were randomized to receive simple advice about discontinuing offending medication, an outpatient detoxification program that included supplementation with prednisone and headache prevention therapy, or inpatient detoxification that similarly included supplementation with prednisone and headache prevention therapy plus intravenous fluids and anti-emetics [30]. When reassessed after two months, outcome was similar among the three groups with no significant differences on any outcome measure (Figure 3). Therefore, initial treatment for most patients with medication overuse headache should include instructions for medication withdrawal.

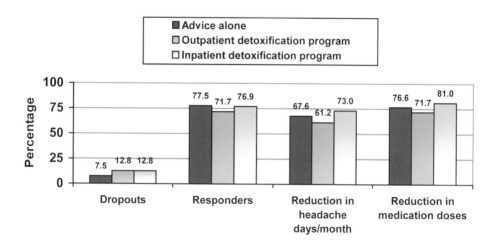

Figure 3 Two-month outcome following medication withdrawal. Responders were defined as having headache resolution or a reduction in headache frequency to <15 days per month plus a reduction in medication use to <10 days per month. (Based on Rossi 2006.)

One month after completing medication withdrawal, headache diaries should be reassessed to determine the current headache pattern, which is often different from the pre-withdrawal pattern. Medication withdrawal alone is effective for nearly half of patients with medication overuse headache. A total of 216 patients with medication overuse headache treated with medication withdrawal were maintained medication-free for two months and reassessed (Figure 4) [31]. Headache frequency was reduced for 45% and unchanged for 48%. Interestingly, despite frequently verbalized fears by patients that medication withdrawal will result in incapacitating headaches, only 7% reported headache aggravation. These data support the benefits of medication withdrawal. This study further highlights that, despite patients' beliefs that overused medications are controlling their headaches, excessive acute medications tend to be ineffective; hence, few patients experienced worsening after drug cessation.

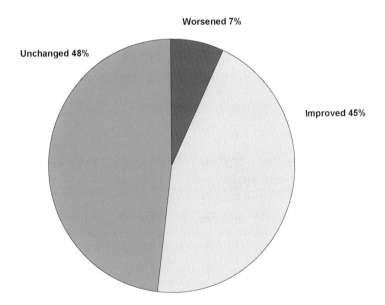

Figure 4 Two-month outcome after medication withdrawal. The pie chart shows the percentage of patients in each post-treatment category. All patients were medication-free following withdrawal. (Based on Zeeberg 2006.)

Post-treatment diaries will help determine if residual headaches should be managed with infrequent acute therapy or daily prevention. Patients continuing to report frequent headaches after medication withdrawal are candidates for prevention therapy. Because the overuse of acute therapies not only results in increased headache activity but also reduces the effectiveness of standard prevention therapy, patients will typically experience a superior response to prevention therapies after medication withdrawal. One study treating patients with medication overuse headache reported using preventive therapy in 47% of patients [32]. Subsequent reduction in headache frequency was similar between those patients who reported a previous non-response to prevention medications (49% decrease) and those who had never used prevention therapy (56% decrease). Therefore, it is often worthwhile to try new prevention therapy, as well as re-try those medications that were previously ineffective while overusing acute therapy in patients after medication withdrawal who still report frequent headaches.

Post-trauma headache

Post-trauma headaches are typically transient. During the first few weeks of treatment, severe headaches with migrainous features are often present, with severity decreasing over time to be more typical of tension-type headaches. Treatment regimens for patients with post-trauma headache should be similar to those used for migraine, with frequent headaches treated with prevention therapy and infrequent, severe episodes managed with acute therapy (see below).

Medication use should be closely monitored in patients with post-trauma headache to prevent the development of excessive use of acute therapies and the consequent conversion of temporary post-trauma headaches into recalcitrant medication overuse headaches. Furthermore, patients who experience worsening or progression of post-traumatic headache symptoms will require reassessment to rule out the presence of ongoing pathology, such as a subdural hematoma.

Treating migraine

Treatment selection for migraine depends on headache frequency and severity (Figure 5). Patients who are not overusing acute care medication but have frequent mild headaches and infrequent severe headaches (e.g., combined migraine and tension-type headache) may benefit from both preventive and acute therapy.

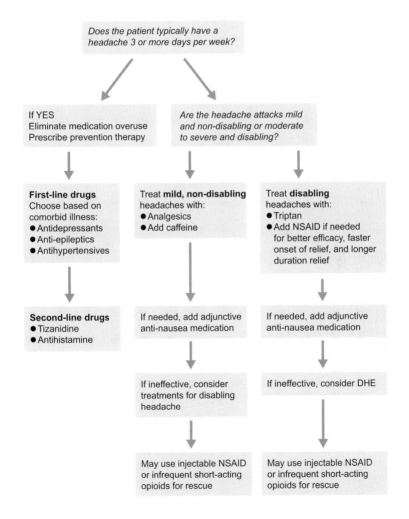

Figure 5 Migraine treatment algorithm. NSAID=non-steroidal anti-inflammatory drug.

When to treat

In general, patients typically experience better headache relief if they treat their symptoms when the severity is milder. Therefore, patients should be advised to treat early during a headache episode rather than waiting until symptoms become severe and disabling.

Allodynia is an important clinical marker of more recalcitrant migraine. Once patients develop allodynia during a migraine episode (e.g., hair hurts, pain with wearing glasses or earrings, or sensitivity of the skin to touch, pressure, heat, or cold), their effective response to acute medication is significantly impaired. For example, sumatriptan treatment effectively resolved migraine episodes in 93% of patients treated before allodynia occurred compared with only 15% after developing allodynia [33].

Interestingly, migraine patients with an acute attack and established allodynia that fail to respond to a triptan have been shown to respond to intravenous ketorolac [34]. Those patients failing to respond to ketorolac shared a pattern of a long history of opioid use. Prolonged exposure to opioids was postulated to activate central mechanisms that impaired reponse to acute migraine drugs. These data suggest the following recommendations:

◆ triptans should be administered early during a migraine attack - prior to the onset of clinical allodynia;
◆ acute treatment after allodynia has already been established or as rescue therapy should include cyclo-oxygenase 1 and 2 inhibitors, such as ketorolac or indomethacin;
◆ opioids should be limited in migraine patients.

Treating tension-type headaches

Similar to migraine, infrequent tension-type headache should be treated with acute care therapies, while more frequent episodes may require prevention treatment. In general, the same acute and preventive therapies that are effective for migraine are also effective for problematic tension-type headaches [35]. For example, sumatriptan and rizatriptan have demonstrated efficacy in clinical trials against both migraine headaches and moderate to severe tension-type headache episodes [36, 37]. In general, however, tension-type headaches are milder than migraine so that analgesics are more appropriate therapy. Tension-type headaches are often frequent and necessitate prevention treatment. Standard headache prevention therapy (with the exception of valproate) are similarly effective for migraine or tension-type headaches.

Treating cluster headache

The intensity of each individual cluster headache attack is so severe that therapy must focus on prevention. Acute therapies are reserved for rescue treatment. Due to the brief nature of cluster attacks, most acute therapies will not become effective before the attack will have spontaneously resolved. Specific treatment recommendations vary, depending on the duration of the cluster episode: episodic versus chronic. Episodic cluster attacks last for ≥7 days, with pain-free periods between clusters of ≥1 month. Episodic cluster attacks typically last about six weeks. Chronic cluster attacks, conversely, are associated with a cluster period lasting >1 year, with any pain-free periods during that year lasting <1 month.

Episodic cluster headache should have preventive therapy initiated at the first occurrence of an attack during a cluster period, with therapy continuing for the expected duration of the cluster cycle (Table 10). Anecdotally, some recalcitrant episodic cluster patients may experience headache prevention from a bedtime dose of a long-acting triptan, such as frovatriptan [38]. If patients are initially diagnosed when a cluster period has already reached peak severity, treatment with a short course of steroids is usually necessary. Plans should be made at that time, however, for initiation of preventive therapy at the start of the next cluster cycle.

Table 10 Treatment of episodic cluster headache.

Preventive therapy: onset of cluster
- Discontinuation of nicotine and alcohol during cluster

- 240-480mg/day verapamil for 6 weeks

- 2-8mg/day methysergide for 6 weeks

Preventive therapy: cluster at maximum intensity at time of treatment initiation
- Prednisone 10-60mg/day for 1 week

Rescue therapy
- 6mg subcutaneous sumatriptan

- 100% O_2 7L/minute for 10 minutes by face mask

- Intranasal butorphanol

Chronic cluster has no or only brief headache-free periods, necessitating treatment with daily, ongoing, preventive therapy (Table 11).

Table 11 Chronic cluster treatment.

Preventive therapy
- Discontinuation of nicotine and alcohol

- 240-480mg/day verapamil

- 250-1000mg/day valproic acid

- 900-1800mg/day gabapentin

Rescue therapy
- 100% O_2 7L/minute for 10 minutes by face mask

Both episodic and chronic cluster headache treatments are not expected to reduce the severity of individual headache attacks. Successful cluster therapy typically results in reduced frequency and duration of headaches. For this reason, a reduction in headache frequency is the main goal of cluster headache therapy.

Nicotine and alcohol are both linked to cluster headache. For example, both cigarette smoking and daily alcohol consumption were reported more frequently in patients with cluster headache (N=374) compared with the general population (Figure 6) [39]. A recent survey of 316 patients with chronic cluster headache similarly identified current or former smoking in 87% of patients [40]. Interestingly, prolonged childhood second-hand smoke exposure has also been linked to the development of cluster headache in adult non-smokers with cluster headache [41]. Anecdotally, patients on occasion report cluster headache improvement after smoking cessation. An internet-based survey of cluster headache sufferers, however, reported that 74% had discontinued nicotine, with headache relief occurring in only 3% [42]. Alcohol consumption reliably triggers a headache attack during the cluster period. Therefore, most cluster headache patients will learn to avoid alcohol during their clusters.

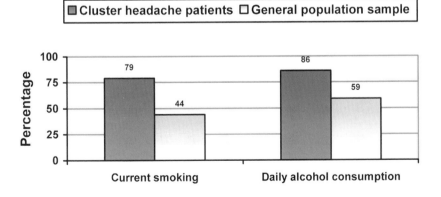

Figure 6 Smoking and daily alcohol use in cluster headache. (Based on Manzoni 1999.)

When to refer

The European Headache Foundation has published headache treatment recommendations, including circumstances suggesting referral to a headache specialist [43]. These guidelines suggest that most cases of migraine and medication overuse headache can be well managed by primary care. Referral to a specialist is suggested when:

◆   a secondary headache disorder is suspected;
◆   the diagnosis is uncertain;
◆   the patient describes an aura that is prolonged (>1 hour), associated with motor weakness, occurs without associated headache, or was precipitated by treatment with oral contraceptives;
◆   comorbid conditions are present, including cardiovascular disease;
◆   the patient has failed the usual treatment options;
◆   the patient is diagnosed with a cluster headache.

Conclusions

Headache medications are divided into acute drugs for relieving individual headache episodes in progress and preventive therapy to reduce the risk for future headaches occurring. Appropriate selection and administration of acute and preventive therapies maximize achieving effective headache control. The choice of acute treatment depends on headache severity and the presence of associated nausea and/or vomiting. A preventive therapy preference is frequently dependent on the presence of comorbid illness. Emerging therapies are currently under testing as both headache acute and preventive therapies.

Key Summary

◆ Headache treatment selection depends on: headache frequency, symptom severity, and comorbid illness.

◆ Acute headache treatments should be used for infrequent headaches, with regular dosing limited to a maximum of three days per week.

◆ Prevention therapy should be used in patients with frequent headache who are not overusing acute medications.

◆ The initial treatment for medication overuse headache is acute drug withdrawal.

◆ Acute migraine treatments include analgesics plus caffeine for mild attacks, triptans for disabling headaches, and anti-emetics for headaches with associated nausea or vomiting.

◆ New, innovative therapies targeting the calcitonin gene-related peptide and other receptors or unique headache mechanisms, including cortical spreading depression, may offer novel treatment options.

◆ Cluster headache treatment focuses on attack prevention.

References

1. Peroutka SJ, Lyon JA, Swarbrick J, Liption RB, Kolodner K, Goldstein J. Efficacy of diclofenac sodium softgel 100mg with or without caffeine 100mg in migraine without aura: a randomized, double-blind, crossover study. *Headache* 2004; 44: 136-141.
2. Evers S, Áfra J, Frese A, *et al.* EFNS guideline on the drug treatment of migraine - report of an EFNS task force. *Eur J Neurol* 2006; 13: 560-572.

3. Ferrari MD, Goadsby PJ, Roon KI, Lipton RB. Triptans (serotonin, 5-HT1B/1D agonists) in migraine: detailed results and methods of a meta-analysis of 53 trials. *Cephalalgia* 2002; 22: 633-658.

4. Mathew NT, Kailasam J, Gentry P, Chernyshev O. Treatment of nonresponders to oral sumatriptan with zolmitriptan and rizatriptan: a comparative open trial. *Headache* 2000; 40: 464-465.

5. Diener HC, Dodick DW, Goadsby PJ, *et al*. Identification of negative predictors of pain-free response to triptans: analysis of the eletriptan database. *Cephalalgia* 2007; 28: 35-40.

6. Krymchantowski AV, Barbosa JS. Rizatriptan combined with rofecoxib vs. rizatriptan for the acute treatment of migraine: an open label pilot study. *Cephalalgia* 2002; 22: 309-312.

7. Brandes JL, Kudrow D, Stark SR, *et al*. Sumatriptan-naproxen for acute treatment of migraine: a randomized trial. *JAMA* 2007; 297:1443-1454.

8. Jones J, Pack S, Chun E. Intramuscular prochlorperazine versus metoclopramide as single-agent therapy for the treatment of acute migraine headache. *Ann Emerg Med* 1996; 14: 262-264.

9. Friedman BW, Esses D, Soloranzo C, *et al*. A randomized controlled trial of prochlorperazine versus metoclopramide for treatment of acute migraine. *Ann Emerg Med*, in press.

10. Gruppo LQ. Intravenous Zofran for headache. *J Emerg Med* 2006; 31: 228-229.

11. Salvatore CA, Hershey JC, Corcoran HA, *et al*. Pharmacological characterization of MK-0974 [N-[(3R,6S)-6-(2,3-difluorophenyl)-2-oxo-1-(2,2,2-trifluoroethyl)azepan-3-yl]-4-(2-oxo-2,3-dihydro-1H-imidazo[4,5-b]pyridin-1-yl)piperidine-1-carboxamide], a potent and orally active calcitonin gene-related peptide receptor antagonist for the treatment of migraine. *J Pharmacol Exp Ther* 2008; 324: 416-421.

12. Ho TW, Mannix LK, Fan X, *et al*. Randomized controlled trial of an oral CGRP receptor antagonist, MK-0974, in acute treatment of migraine. *Neurology* 2008; 70: 1304-1312.

13. Vause C, Bowen E, Spierings E, Durham P. Effect of carbon dioxide on calcitonin gene-related peptide secretion from trigeminal neurons. *Headache* 2007; 47:1385-1397.

14. Spierings G. Abortive treatment of migraine headache with non-inhaled, intranasal carbon dioxide: a randomized, double-blind, placebo-controlled, parallel-group study. *Headache* 2005; 45: 809.

15. Gunthorpe MJ, Szallasi A. Peripheral TRPV1 receptors as targets for drug development: new molecules and mechanisms. *Curr Pharm Des* 2008; 14: 32-41.

16. De Alba J, Clayton NM, Collins SD, *et al*. GW274150, a novel and highly selective inhibitor of the inducible isoform of nitric oxide synthase (iNOS), shows analgesic effects in rat models of inflammatory and neuropathic pain. *Pain* 2006; 120: 170-181.

17. Siegel SJ, O'Neill C, Dubé LM, *et al*. A unique iontophoretic patch for optimal transdermal delivery of sumatriptan. *Pharm Res* 2007; 24: 1919-1926.

18. Mathew NT, Rapoport A, Saper J, *et al*. Efficacy of gabapentin in migraine prophylaxis. *Headache* 2001; 41: 119-128.

19. Brighina F, Palermo A, Aloisio A, *et al*. Levetiracetam in the prophylaxis of migraine with aura: a 6-month open-label study. *Clin Neuropharmacol* 2006; 29: 338-342.

20. Saper JR, Lake AE, Cantrell DT, Winner PK, White JR. Chronic daily headache prophylaxis with tizanidine: a double-blind, placebo-controlled, multicenter outcome study. *Headache* 2002; 42: 470-482.

21. D'Amico D, Lanteri-Minet M. Migraine preventive therapy: selection of appropriate patients and general principles of management. *Expert Rev Neurother* 2006; 6: 1147-1157.

22. Gupta P, Singh S, Goyal V, Shukla G, Behari M. Low-dose topiramate versus lamotrigine in migraine prophylaxis (the Lotolamp study). *Headache* 2007; 47: 402-412.

23. Togha M, Ashrafian H, Tajik P. Open-label trial of cinnarizine in migraine prophylaxis. *Headache* 2006; 46: 498-502.

24. Rossi P, Fiermonte G, Pierelli F. Cinnarizine in migraine prophylaxis: efficacy, tolerability and predictive factors for therapeutic responsiveness. An open-label pilot trial. *Funct Neurol* 2003; 18: 155-159.

25. Tomkins GE, Jackson JL, O'Malley PG, Balden E, Santoro JE. Treatment of chronic headache with antidepressants: a meta-analysis. *Am J Med* 2001; 111: 54-63.

26. Saper JR, Lake AE, Hamel RL, *et al.* Daily scheduled opioids for intractable head pain: long-term observations of a treatment program. *Neurology* 2004; 62: 1687-1694.

27. Goadsby PJ, Ferrari MD, Olesen J, Mills JG. Double-blind placebo-controlled trial of tonabersat in the preventive management of migraine. *Cephalalgia* 2007; 27: 1195-1196.

28. Schwedt TJ, Dodick DW, Hentz J, Trentman TL, Zimmerman RS. Occipital nerve stimulation for chronic headache - long-term safety and efficacy. *Cephalalgia* 2007; 27: 153-157.

29. http://www.fda.gov/cder/drug/InfoSheets/HCP/antiepilepticsHCP.htm. (Accessed February 2008).

30. Rossi P, Di Lorenzo C, Faroni J, Cesarino F, Nappi G. Advice alone vs. structured detoxification programmes for medication overuse headache: a prospective, randomized, open-label trial in transformed migraine patients with low medical needs. *Cephalalgia* 2006; 26: 1097-1105.

31. Zeeberg P, Olesen J, Jensen R. Probable medication-overuse headache. The effect of a 2-month drug-free period. *Neurology* 2006; 66: 1894-1898.

32. Zeeberg P, Olesen J, Jensen R. Discontinuation of medication overuse in headache patients: recovery of therapeutic responsiveness. *Cephalalgia* 2006; 26: 1192-1198.

33. Burstein R, Collins B, Jakubowski M. Defeating migraine pain with triptans: a race against the development of cutaneous allodynia. *Ann Neurol* 2004; 55: 19-26.

34. Jakubowski M, Levy D, Goor-Aryeh I, *et al.* Terminating migraine with allodynia and ongoing central sensitization using parenteral administration of COX 1/COX 2 inhibitors. *Headache* 2005; 45: 850-861.

35. Marcus DA. Migraine and tension-type headaches: the questionable validity of current classification systems. *Clin J Pain* 1992; 8: 28-36.

36. Lipton RB, Stewart WF, Cady R, *et al.* Sumatriptan for the range of headaches in migraine sufferers: results of the Spectrum Study. *Headache* 2000; 40: 783-791.

37. Allen C, Cady R, Lines C, McCarroll K. Effect of rizatriptan in the spectrum of headache. *Headache* 2001; 41: 607-608.

38. Siow HC, Pozo-Rosich P, Silberstein SD. Frovatriptan for the treatment of cluster headache. *Cephalalgia* 2004; 24: 1045-1048.

39. Manzoni GC. Cluster headache and lifestyle: remarks on a population of 374 male patients. *Cephalalgia* 1999; 19: 88-94.

40. Donnet A, Lanteri-Minet M, Guegan-Massardier E, *et al.* Chronic cluster headache: a French clinical descriptive study. *J Neurol Neurosurg Psychiatry* 2007; 78: 1354-1358.

41. Rozen TD. Childhood exposure to second-hand tobacco smoke and the development of cluster headache. *Headache* 2005; 45: 393-394.

42. Klapper JA, Klapper A, Voss T. The misdiagnosis of cluster headache: a nonclinic, population-based, internet survey. *Headache* 2000; 40: 730-735.

43. Steiner TJ, Paemeleire K, Jensen R, *et al.* European principles of management of common headache disorders in primary care. *J Headache Pain* 2007; 8: S3-S21

Chapter 6
Headache comorbidity

Introduction

Separate and independent disorders often occur simultaneously in the same patient. When this happens, healthcare providers and patients often want to know if one disorder caused the other, if the two conditions are related, or if the two conditions are occurring by chance alone. For example, patients with diabetes often develop retinal, heart, and kidney dysfunction. These disorders are directly caused by the underlying primary disorder of diabetes. Patients with schizophrenia, conversely, have an increased risk of also experiencing a mood disorder as a comorbid condition. Finally, a patient with hypercholesterolemia may develop bursitis as a separate and unrelated disorder.

Comorbidity is often described using an odds ratio (OR). This statistical tool is used to compare the probability of a certain event occurring simultaneously in two separate groups. A ratio is calculated comparing those with versus those without the event under study. When there is an equal chance that both groups will have a condition, the OR is one. This occurs when two conditions are co-occurring, their association based on chance alone. An OR greater than one means the two conditions occur together more frequently than would be predicted by chance. An OR less than one shows that the conditions occur together less commonly than predicted by chance alone.

The significance of the OR is understood by evaluating the 95% confidence interval (abbreviated CI). The confidence interval gives a likely range of possible values that would be compatible with the data. The endpoints of the confidence interval are called confidence limits. Significant values are those for which the 95% CI does not include the number 1.0.

Comorbidity can also be described using relative risk (RR), the proportion of people with a condition in one group compared with a control group. No effect is shown when the RR is one, while a complete association relationship is described when the RR is zero. The significance of RR is similarly defined using 95% CI. RR can also be described using the hazard ratio (HR), which estimates RR using survival analyses. A HR of one means that the conditions are equivalent. A HR of two means that an event occurred in twice as many individuals with one condition versus another. Conversely, half as many people are affected with the HR of 0.5.

A face-to-face household survey reported the occurrence of a wide range of medical conditions in adults with and without headache [1]. The prevalence in each group is shown in Figure 1, while calculated ORs with

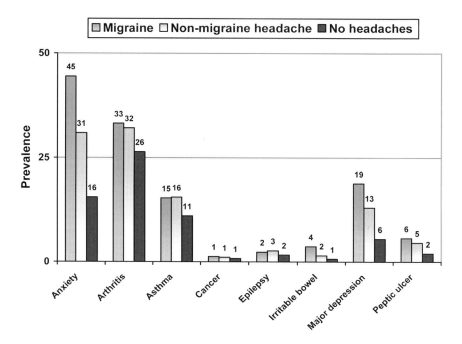

Figure 1 Prevalence of conditions in adults with frequent or severe migraine or non-migraine headache during the previous 12 months or no headache. (Based on Saunders 2008.)

Table 1 ORs (95% CI) for the occurrence of a health condition. Significant relationships are highlighted. (Based on Saunders 2008.)

Health condition	No headache	Headache	
		Migraine	Not migraine
Anxiety	1.00	**3.1 (2.5-3.9)**	**2.0 (1.6-2.6)**
Arthritis	1.00	**2.2 (1.5-3.2)**	**2.0 (1.4-2.8)**
Asthma	1.00	**1.3 (0.7-2.2)**	1.3 (0.9-2.0)
Cancer	1.00	3.3 (0.8-13.7)	2.3 (0.8-7.1)
Epilepsy	1.00	1.0 (0.5-2.0)	1.4 (0.6-2.9)
Irritable bowel	1.00	**3.8 (1.3-11.4)**	1.8 (0.5-6.1)
Major depression	1.00	**2.8 (2.0-3.9)**	**2.1 (1.5-3.1)**
Peptic ulcer	1.00	**2.5 (1.5-4.1)**	2.4 (1.0-5.3)

a 95% CI in Table 1 help to demonstrate which numerical differences in prevalence between a headache group versus no headache sample is more likely to represent a greater than chance relationship or comorbidity. These data show a relationship between several conditions and chronic headache, highlighted in Table 1.

Cardiovascular disease and stroke

Chest pain and cardiovascular risk factors

Reports of chest pain often cause alarm as a forecaster of cardiac pathology. Chest pain was a more frequently identified symptom in patients with migraine compared with those without migraine (21% vs. 14%, P<0.01) in a retrospective database review [2]. Cardiovascular events, however, were not convincingly linked to the diagnosis of migraine in this analysis, questioning the significance of increased chest pain as a symptom.

Special concern about cardiovascular disease is warranted in headache patients, as cardiovascular risk factors have also been linked to the diagnosis of migraine. The population-based Genetic Epidemiology of Migraine study in the Netherlands evaluated cardiovascular risk factors in 5755 adults, based on a history of migraine or not [3]. Significantly increased risk factors in migraineurs are shown in Figure 2. Risk was more often associated with migraine with aura than migraine without aura. For example, the Framingham ten-year risk of myocardial infarction or coronary heart disease death was elevated in migraine with aura (OR=4.01 [95% CI=1.1-15.0]), with substantially lower numbers for migraine without aura (OR=1.84 [95% CI=0.7-5.0]).

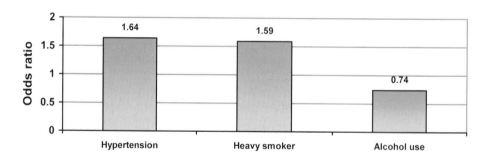

Figure 2 Odds ratios for the prevalence of cardiovascular risk factors and migraine.

Cerebrovascular accidents

In general, patients with migraine with aura are considered to have a significantly increased risk of stroke compared with non-headache controls, while migraine without aura is not associated with an increased risk. The relationship between migraine and stroke was assessed in the large, prospective Women's Health Study (N=39,876) in which apparently healthy female healthcare workers without cardiovascular disease were followed for an average of nine years for the occurrence of cerebrovascular accidents and other events [4]. Ischemic stroke was significantly more likely to occur in women also reporting migraine with aura (Table 2).

Table 2 Relationship between migraine and stroke, HR (95% CI), adjusted for other cardiovascular risk factors. Significant relationships are highlighted. (Based on Kurth 2005.)

Stroke type	No migraine	Migraine		
		Any	Aura	No aura
Any stroke	1.00	1.23 (0.90-1.69)	**1.54 (1.02-2.35)**	1.01 (0.65-1.56)
Ischemic	1.00	1.36 (0.97-1.92)	**1.73 (1.10-2.71)**	1.11 (0.69-1.78)
Hemorrhagic	1.00	0.78 (0.33-1.82)	0.94 (0.29-3.00)	0.67 (0.21-2.14)

Even though cerebrovascular accidents are more likely in patients with migraine with aura, stroke is rarely seen in these patients because the overall risk of stroke in young adults is very low. The Women's Health Study reported above, for example, estimated there would be nine ischemic strokes per 10,000 women annually among those with no migraine versus 12 strokes per 10,000 women annually among those with migraine [4]. Understanding this risk, however, is important to try to minimize additional modifiable risk factors, such as hypertension, obesity, hypercholesterolemia, and cigarette smoking in patients with migraine with aura. Furthermore, oral contraceptives are often restricted in migraine with aura patients because of the additive risk of ischemic stroke.

Cardiovascular disease

The Women's Health Study described above similarly linked migraine with aura and ischemic cardiovascular disease [5]. Migraine with aura was associated with an increased risk for non-fatal and fatal cardiovascular events, while migraine without aura was not (Table 3).

Table 3 Relationship between migraine and cardiovascular events, OR (95% CI), adjusted for other cardiovascular risk factors. Significant relationships are highlighted. (Based on Kurth 2006.)

Ischemic event	No migraine	Migraine	
		Aura	No aura
Major cardiovascular event	1.00	**2.15 (1.58-2.92)**	1.23 (0.88-1.73)
Angina	1.00	**1.71 (1.16-2.53)**	1.12 (0.75-1.66)
Myocardial infarction	1.00	**2.08 (1.30-3.31)**	1.22 (0.73-2.05)
Coronary revascularization	1.00	**1.74 (1.23-2.46)**	0.98 (0.67-1.42)
Cardiovascular death	1.00	**2.33 (1.21-4.51)**	1.06 (0.46-2.45)

The Physicians' Health Study likewise prospectively evaluated the relationship between migraine and cardiovascular events in 20,084 apparently healthy male physicians followed for 60 months [6]. Information on type of migraine (with or without aura) was not available for this study. Significant adjusted HRs were reported for patients with migraine versus no migraine for major cardiovascular events (HR=1.24 [95% CI=1.06-1.46]) and myocardial infarction (HR=1.42 [95% CI=1.15-1.77]). Ischemic stroke, coronary revascularization, angina, and cardiovascular death were not more likely in male physicians with migraine. Confidence in lack of risk, however, is limited due to the inability to distinguish risk based on aura, which was important in the analysis of female healthcare workers in the Women's Health Study.

Cardiovascular events and triptans

Triptans constrict both meningeal and coronary arteries *in vitro*; however, they are ten times more potent at the meningeal than coronary vessels [7, 8]. Both triptans and ergotamines are restricted in patients with ischemic heart disease, a stroke history, or uncontrolled hypertension as they constrict coronary vessels in the laboratory. Because the degree of constriction is small, triptans and ergotamines may be used in healthy migraineurs [9].

Intravenous and subcutaneous sumatriptan cause an increase in systemic and pulmonary artery pressures and vascular resistance, without a change in cardiac output [10, 11]. Coronary artery diameter is reduced by 13% ten minutes after intravenous injection, 16% ten minutes after subcutaneous injection, and 17% 30 minutes after subcutaneous injection. Myocardial perfusion after injection of 6mg sumatriptan in healthy migraneurs is slightly reduced, although this change is not clinically or statistically significant [12].

Because of the increase in cardiovascular risk factors and events in migraineurs, cardiovascular events occurring in patients treated with triptans may be related to treatment, underlying risk, or unrelated factors. Jhee *et al* reported the incidence of cardiovascular events in subjects enrolled in a triptan trial who had received placebo only [13]. Electrocardiographic abnormalities were identified in 67% of these placebo-treated subjects. This study highlights the importance of comparing cardiovascular monitors in placebo or non-treatment populations to avoid overdiagnosis of cardiac abnormalities with treatment.

Headache experts recently summarized data from large observational studies that failed to show a link between triptan use and a risk of stroke or myocardial infarction [14]. Overuse of triptans was similarly not linked to the increased occurrence of vascular events, while overuse of ergotamine did increase risk (OR=2.55 [95% CI=1.22-5.36]).

Patent foramen ovale (PFO) and migraine

In the general population, about one in every five adults has a patent foramen ovale (PFO). Migraineurs, especially those with migraine with aura, have an increased prevalence of PFO. A case-controlled study, for example, showed a significantly higher prevalence of PFO in migrainuers versus controls (P<0.01), with a PFO identified in 67% of migraineurs with aura, 47% of migraineurs without aura, and 22% of controls [15].

Preliminary reports linked repair of PFOs or atrial septal defects (ASDs) with a marked reduction in the severity and frequency of migraine attacks in patients with either migraine with or without aura [16-18]. Researchers speculated that chemicals that would normally be filtered by the lungs may trigger migraines. Another possibility is that there may be a genetic link between heart defects and migraine. Several studies, however, have also reported worsening of migraine or the development of new migraines after these repairs [17, 19].

In order to more carefully study the effect of PFO repair on migraine, 147 migraine with aura patients were randomized to PFO closure or sham surgery in the Migraine Intervention with STARFlex Technology (MIST) trial [20]. Researchers hoped to replicate previous, uncontrolled treatment reports of a high percentage of migraine patients experiencing headache resolution after PFO repair. Migraine resolved in only 4% with either actual or sham surgery in the MIST trial. The number of days with headache over a three-month period decreased similarly for both groups (about a 30% reduction). Headache severity likewise decreased for both groups by about 12%. There were no significant between-group differences, failing to show benefit from this procedure as a migraine therapy.

Epilepsy

Comorbidity between migraine and epilepsy is controversial. While studies have historically shown about a two-fold increased prevalence of migraine in those with epilepsy, recently studies have failed to confirm an increased occurrence of headache in individuals with seizure disorders [21]. While a relationship between migraine in general and epilepsy is questionable, a relationship appears to exist for migraine with aura and epilepsy [21]. Large-scale studies are needed to clarify this relationship.

Fibromyalgia

Fibromyalgia is a chronic pain condition with widespread body pain, tenderness to palpation of tenderpoint areas, and constitutional symptoms. In 1990, the American College of Rheumatology (ACR) established specific criteria to allow identification of fibromyalgia as a unique pain syndrome, requiring both widespread pain and the presence of at least 11 of 18 painful tenderpoints (Table 4) [22].

Table 4 ACR diagnostic criteria for fibromyalgia. (Based on American College of Rheumatology criteria; Wolfe 1990.)

- Widespread body pain
    - Pain on both left and right sides of the body
    - Pain above and below the waist
    - Axial pain present

- Pain persisting ≥3 months

- ≥11 of 18 tenderpoints painful to 4kg pressure

Tenderpoints are predetermined areas throughout the body that tend to be painful with pressure in patients with fibromyalgia (Figure 3). Positive tenderpoints discriminate between fibromyalgia patients and other pain patients when using a cut-off score of at least two on a 0-10 severity scale (0 = pressure only with no pain; 10 = excruciating pain) after the application of 4kg of pressure [23]. Digital palpation more effectively discriminates fibromyalgia patients than dolorimeter testing, making testing at the bedside easy [22]. Pressing with the thumb results in approximately 4kg of pressure when the nail bed blanches. Higher scores reported for tenderpoints correlate with greater levels of disability [24].

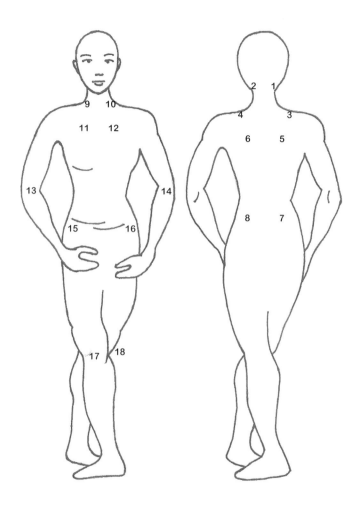

Figure 3 Location of 18 possible fibromyalgia tenderpoints. Location of tenderpoints (right and left): 1 and 2: occiput; 3 and 4: trapezius; 5 and 6: supraspinatus; 7 and 8: gluteal; 9 and 10: lower lateral cervical; 11 and 12: 2nd costochondral junction; 13 and 14: lateral epicondyle; 15 and 16: greater trochanter; 17 and 18: medial knee fat pad. (Reproduced with permission from Springer, © 2005. Marcus DA. *Chronic Pain. A Primary Care Guide to Practical Management.* Humana Press: Totowa, NJ, 2005.)

Patients with fibromyalgia typically describe a variety of additional somatic and psychological complaints, including headache. While fibromyalgia affects 2-3% of the general population, a survey of migraine patients identified fibromyalgia in 17% [25]. Conversely, a survey of 100 fibromyalgia patients seeking treatment for fibromyalgia but not headache were questioned about the occurrence of headache [26]. Three of every four fibromyalgia patients reported having troublesome headache (Figure 4). Interestingly, headache was associated with substantial or severe impact in 84% of these patients, although none was seeking headache treatment. Migraine was the most common diagnosis, occurring in 63% of those patients reporting headache.

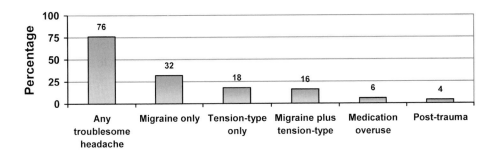

Figure 4 Prevalence of migraine in fibromyalgia patients. (Based on Marcus 2005.)

Mood disorders

Nearly 37,000 Canadians ≥15 years old were evaluated with the World Mental Health Composite Diagnostic Interview in the Canadian Community Health Survey [27]. Migraine was identified as comorbid with a major depressive disorder, bipolar disorder, panic disorder, and social phobia, each of which occurred about twice as often in individuals with migraine (Figure 5).

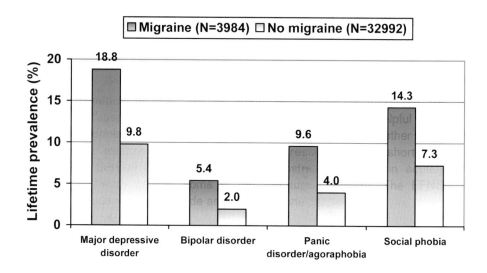

Figure 5 Prevalence of psychiatric disorders. (Based on Jette 2008.)

Patients can be screened for depression and anxiety using a variety of screening tools. Online screening tests can be found at the following websites:

◆ NYU Medical Center site: http://www.med.nyu.edu/psych/screens/;

◆ HealthyPlace.com: http://www.healthyplace.com/site/tests/psychological. asp;

◆ Depression and Bipolar Support Alliance site: http://www.dbsalliance. org/site/PageServer?pagename=about_screening_screeningcenter;

◆ PsychCentral.com: http://psychcentral.com/quizzes/.

Obesity

A survey of consecutive chronic pain patients, 35% of whom had head and neck pain, revealed that pain impact was significantly greater in patients with an increased body mass index (BMI; see Table 5), with patients in increased weight categories reporting an increased frequency of pain-related disability and reduced physical functioning [28]. Evaluations with chronic headache patients have similarly shown a link with frequent migraine and excessive weight. A random survey of adults showed no overall relationship between weight category and the diagnosis of migraine (Figure 6); however, individuals with frequent migraine (episodes occurring 10-14 days per month) were more likely to be overweight or obese (Table 6) [29]. A similar analysis confirmed this relationship in migraine and failed to show a relationship between tension-type headaches and weight, including frequent tension-type headaches [30].

Table 5 Body mass index (BMI) categories (kg/m^2).

- Underweight <18.5

- Normal weight 18.5-24.9

- Overweight 25-29.9

- Obese 30-34.9

- Morbidly obese ≥35

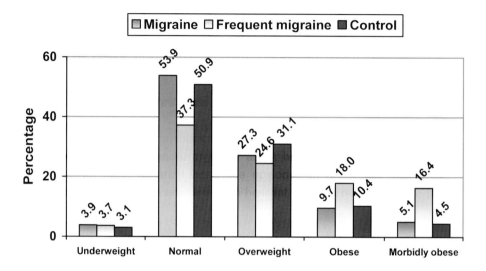

Figure 6 Weight categories in migraine sufferers and controls. (Based on Bigal 2006.)

Table 6 ORs (95% CI) for frequent migraine with abnormal BMI. Significant relationships are highlighted. (Based on Bigal 2006.)

Weight category	Odds of having frequent migraine
Underweight	1.3 (0.6-2.8)
Normal	1.0
Overweight	**1.3 (1.1-1.9)**
Obese	**2.9 (1.9-4.4)**
Morbidly obese	**5.7 (3.6-8.8)**

Gastrointestinal disorders

Although not traditionally linked to headache or migraine, a Norwegian study provided data on headache and gastrointestinal complaints during the preceding 12 months in 43,782 adults [31]. Participants rated the intensity of gastrointestinal symptoms as none, some, or much. ORs in Figure 7 show the risk of having a headache among individuals with 'much' gastrointestinal symptoms compared with 'none.' The OR for no gastrointestinal symptoms was the standard at 1.0. A higher prevalence of any headache, migraine, and non-migraine headache was identified in individuals rating each gastrointestinal symptom as 'much' compared with those without gastrointestinal complaints.

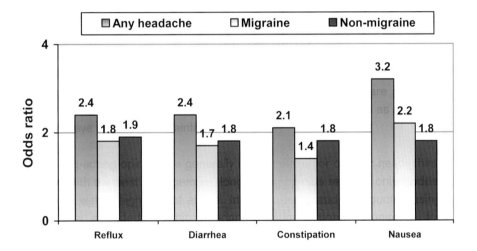

Figure 7 OR of headache among patients with substantial gastrointestinal complaints. The 95% CI did not include 1.0 for any of these ORs. Therefore, all are significant. (Based on Aamodt 2008.)

Conclusions

Both physical and mental disorders occur more commonly in patients with chronic headache disorders than would be expected by chance occurrence. Comorbid conditions include chronic pain disorders, such as arthritis and fibromyalgia, gastrointestinal symptoms, anxiety, and depression. Most comorbidity has been linked to migraine. Migraine is associated with an increased risk of hypertension, chest pain, and cardiovascular disease. The risk of ischemic stroke is almost doubled in women with migraine with aura, although the absolute risk of stroke is still very low. Ischemic cardiovascular events have also been linked to migraine with aura in women and migraine in general in men. Awareness of increased cardiovascular risk should result in a stronger emphasis placed on reducing modifiable risk factors for cardiovascular disease in patients who also have migraine, especially migraine with aura.

Key Summary

◆ Migraine with aura in women is associated with an increased risk of ischemic stroke and cardiovascular disease. Migraine has also been linked to an increased risk of major cardiovascular events and myocardial infarction in men.

◆ PFO can be detected in two of every three migraineurs with aura and half of those without aura. Closing the PFO has not convincingly resulted in headache improvement.

◆ Three of every four patients seeking treatment for fibromyalgia have troublesome headaches, most commonly migraine.

◆ Mood and anxiety disorders occur almost twice as often in those with migraine compared with those without migraine.

◆ Frequent migraine has been linked to an increased risk of being overweight or obese.

◆ Gastrointestinal symptoms, including reflux, diarrhea, constipation, and nausea, occur more commonly in individuals with headache.

◆ Clear comorbidity between migraine and epilepsy has not been established.

References

1. Saunders K, Merikangas K, Low NP, Von Korff M, Kessler RC. Impact of comorbidity on headache-related disability. *Neurology* 2008; 70: 538-547.

2. Sternfeld B, Stang P, Sidney S. Relationship of migraine headaches to experience of chest pain and subsequent risk for myocardial infarction. *Neurology* 1995; 45: 2135-2142.

3. Scher AI, Terwindt GM, Picavet HJ, *et al.* Cardiovascular risk factors and migraine. The GEM population-based study. *Neurology* 2005; 64: 614-620.

4. Kurth T, Slomke MA, Kase CS, *et al.* Migraine, headache, and the risk of stroke in women: a prospective study. *Neurology* 2005; 64: 1020-1026.

5. Kurth T, Gaziano JM, Cook NR, *et al.* Migraine and risk of cardiovascular disease in women. *JAMA* 2006; 296: 283-291.

6. Kurth T, Gaziano JM, Cook NR, *et al.* Migraine and risk of cardiovascular disease in men. *Arch Intern Med* 2007; 167: 795-801.

7. Longmore J, Razzaque Z, Shaw D, Davenport AP, Maguire J, Pickard JD, Schofield WN, Hill RG. Comparison of the vasoconstrictor effects of rizatriptan and sumatriptan in human isolated cranial arteries: immunohistological demonstration of the involvement of 5-HT1B-receptors. *Br J Clin Pharmacol* 1998; 46: 577-582.

8. Parsons AA, Raval P, Smith S, Tilford N, King FD, Kaumann AJ, Hunter J. Effects of the novel high-affinity 5-HT(1B/1D)-receptor ligand frovatriptan in human isolated basilar and coronary arteries. *J Cardiovasc Pharmacol* 1998; 32: 220-224.

9. Maassen van den Brink A, Reekers M, Bax WA, Ferrari MD, Saxena PR. Coronary side-effect potential of current and prospective antimigraine drugs. *Circulation* 1998; 98: 25-30.

10. MacIntyre PD, Bhargava B, Hogg KJ, Gemmill JD, Hillis WS. Effect of subcutaneous sumatriptan, a selective 5HT1 agonist, on the systemic, pulmonary, and coronary circulation. *Circulation* 1993; 87: 401-405.

11. MacIntyre PD, Bharagava B, Hogg KJ, Gemmill JD, Hillis WS. The effect of i.v. sumatriptan, a selective 5-HT1-receptor agonist on central haemodynamics and the coronary circulation. *Br J Clin Pharmacol* 1992; 34: 541-546.

12. Lewis PJ, Barrington SF, Mardsen PK, Maisey MN, Lewis LD. A study of the effects of sumatriptan on myocardial perfusion in healthy female migraineurs using 13NH3 positron emission tomography. *Neurology* 1997; 48: 1542-1550.

13. Jhee SS, Salazar DE, Ford NF, Fulmor IE, Sramek JJ, Cutler NR. Monitoring of acute migraine attacks: placebo response and safety data. *Headache* 1998; 38: 35-38.

14. Diener H, Kurth T, Dodick D. Patent foramen ovale, stroke, and cardiovascular disease in migraine. *Curr Opin Neurol* 2007; 20: 310-319.

15. Tatlidede AD, Oflazoglu B, Celik SE, Anadol U, Forta H. Prevalence of patent foramen ovale in patients with migraine. *Agri* 19: 39-42.

16. Azarbal B, Tobis J, Suh W, *et al.* Association of interatrial shunts and migraine headaches. Impact of transcatheter closure. *J Am Coll Cardiol* 2005; 45: 489-492.

17. Beda RD, Gill EA. Patent foramen ovale: does it play a role in the pathophysiology of migraine headache? *Cardiol Clin* 2005; 23:9 1-96.

18. Reisman M, Christofferson RD, Jesurum J, *et al.* Migraine headache relief after transcatheter closure of patent foramen ovale. *J Am Coll Cardiol* 2005; 45: 493-495.

19. Mortelmans K, Post M, Thijs V, Herroelen L, Budts W. The influence of percutaneous atrial septal defect closure on the occurrence of migraine. *Eur Heart J* 2005; doi:10.1093/eurheart/hei170.

20. Dowson A, Mullen MJ, Peatfield R, *et al.* Migraine Intervention with STARFlex Technology (MIST) trial: a prospective, multicenter, double-blind, sham-controlled trial to evaluate the effectiveness of patient foramen ovale closure with STARFlex septal repair implant to resolve refractory migraine headaches. *Circulation* 2008; 117: 1397-1404.

21. DeSimone R, Ranieri A, Marano E, *et al.* Migraine and epilepsy: clinical and pathophysiological relations. *Neurol Sci* 2007; 28: S150-S155.

22. Wolfe F, Smythe HA, Yunus MB, *et al.* The American College of Rheumatology 1990 criteria for the classification of fibromyalgia: report of the Multicenter Criteria Committee. *Arthritis Rheum* 1990; 33: 160-172.

23. Okifuji A, Turk DC, Sinclair JD, Starz TW, Marcus DA. A standardized manual tender point survey. I. Development and determination of a threshold point for the identification of positive tender points in fibromyalgia syndrome. *J Rheumatol* 1997; 24: 377-83.

24. Lundberg G, Gerdle B. Tender point scores and their relations to signs of mobility, symptoms, and disability in female home care personnel and the prevalence of fibromyalgia. *J Rheumatol* 2002; 29: 603-613.

25. Ifergane G, Buskila D, Simiseshvely N, Zeev K, Cohen H. Prevalence of fibromyalgia syndrome in migraine patients. *Cephalalgia* 2006; 26: 451-6.

26. Marcus DA, Bernstein C, Rudy TE. Fibromyalgia and headache: an epidemiological study supporting migraine as part of the fibromyalgia syndrome. *Clin Rheumatol* 2005; 24: 595-601.

27. Jette N, Patten S, Williams J, Becker W, Wiebe S. Comorbidity of migraine and psychiatric disorders - a national population-based study. *Headache* 2008; 48: 501-516.

28. Marcus DA. Obesity and the impact of chronic pain. *Clin J Pain* 2004; 20: 186-191.

29. Bigal ME, Liberman JN, Lipton RB. Obesity and migraine. A population study. *Neurology* 2006; 66: 545-550.

30. Bigal ME, Tsang A, Loder E, *et al.* Body mass index and episodic headaches. A population-based study. *Arch Intern Med* 2007; 167: 1964-1970.

31. Aamodt AH, Stovner LJ, Hagen K, Zwart J. Comorbidity of headache and gastrointestinal complaints. The Head-HUNT Study. *Cephalalgia* 2008; 28: 144-151.

Chapter 7

Complementary and alternative therapies

Introduction

Complementary and alternative medicine are commonly used for the treatment of a wide variety of health symptoms as well as preventive health maintenance (Table 1). As the names imply, complementary medicine is designed to supplement conventional therapy, while alternative therapies often provide an approach that differs from and replaces traditional medical care. The use of complementary and alternative medicine varies across the world, with specific therapies utilized also varying by region (Figure 1) [1-5].

A variety of complementary and alternative therapies have been tested for headache treatment. Therapies can be divided into good efficacy (similar to traditional medications), moderate efficacy (less effective than traditional medications), and ineffective (Table 2). For example, the European Federation of Neurological Sciences recommends Petasites (butterbur) as second-line preventive therapy after effective medications such as beta-blockers, calcium channel blockers, and neurostabilizing anti-epileptics, with coenzyme Q10, magnesium, riboflavin, and Tanacetum (feverfew) recommended as third-line prevention. Some therapies, like hypnosis, have demonstrated good efficacy, although studies available for review predate the current classification system for headache, limiting interpretation [6].

Table 1 Examples of complementary and alternative therapy.

- Acupuncture
- Aromatherapy
- Biofeedback
- Chiropractic medicine
- Herbal medicine
- Homeopathy
- Hypnosis
- Massage
- Naturopathy
- Nutritional therapy
- Reflexology
- Spiritual healing
- Tai Chi
- Traditional Chinese medicine
- Yoga

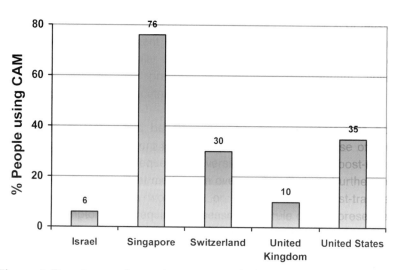

Figure 1 Prevalence of complementary and alternative medicine (CAM) use during the preceding 12 months. (Based on Niskar 2007, Lim 2005, Rössler 2007, Thomas 2004, Tindle 2005.)

Table 2 Complementary and alternative medicines for headache.

Effective	Moderately effective	Ineffective
Biofeedback	Feverfew (*Tanacetum parthenium*)	Acupuncture
Butterbur (*Petasites*)	Coenzyme Q10	Botulinum toxin injections
Relaxation	Diet	
Stress management	Exercise	
	Hypnosis	
	Intraoral appliance	
	Magnesium	
	Physical therapy	
	Massage	
	Riboflavin	
	Sleep hygiene	
	Smoking cessation	

Treating healthcare providers need to be knowledgeable about complementary and alternative therapies. A recent survey revealed that 62% of patients expect to receive complementary and alternative medicine as part of their routine medical visits, while only 30% of doctors shared this view [7].

Effective therapies

Highly effective non-medication therapies can be used as first-line treatment and may sometimes be used as prevention monotherapy. Efficacy is enhanced by combining effective medication and non-medication therapies [8]. In some cases, once headaches have been well controlled for six months, preventive medications can be tapered, with headache control maintenance achieved by continuing non-medication therapies [9-11]. In a recent study of 818 adults with migraine from 21 countries in Europe and the Middle East, open-label prevention therapy with topiramate resulted in a substantial reduction in headache frequency [12].

After six months of open-label treatment, patients were randomly assigned to continue topiramate or switch to placebo. Benefits were maintained after six months of double-blind treatment with either continued topiramate or placebo, although there was a small but significant increase in headache frequency with placebo (P<0.0001) (Figure 2). These data support attempting to taper prevention therapy after six months of effective treatment. Patients should continue non-medication therapies during this time to help maximize long-term maintenance of headache control.

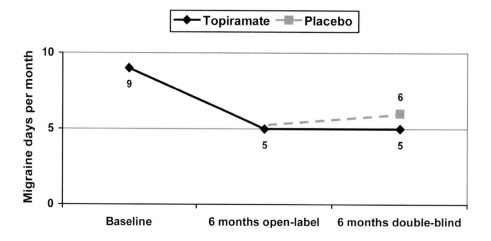

Figure 2 Long-term headache control after discontinuation of effective headache prevention medication. (Based on Diener 2007.)

Relaxation and biofeedback

Relaxation techniques, including biofeedback, are among the most effective preventive therapies for migraine and tension-type headaches (Table 3). Biofeedback relies on external monitors to indicate that the appropriate level of relaxation has been reached, providing patient feedback with complex computerized monitors of muscle contraction with graphic displays or simple hand-held thermometers designed to demonstrate a few degree increase in hand temperature when relaxation has been achieved. No single relaxation technique is superior to the others, although some patients find that they prefer using one technique. Biofeedback is traditionally taught by a trained therapist over 12 treatment sessions, although similar efficacy is achieved using a minimal therapist contact approach with about five or six treatment sessions and home practice between supervised training appointments. Skills should be practiced daily during training. Once patients have mastered these skills, they no longer have to use them regularly, but may use them as needed.

Table 3 Relaxation techniques.

- Visual imagery

- Deep breathing techniques

- Progressive muscle relaxation

- Biofeedback

Relaxation or biofeedback techniques have a similar efficacy to standard migraine preventive medications, without the associated side effects. About 50-80% of patients motivated to learn these techniques experience relief [13-15]. In a recent study, benefits from six months of training with relaxation with biofeedback versus propranolol were compared in 192 migraine patients [15]. Headache frequency, duration, and severity were significantly improved with either treatment ($P<0.05$), with no between-group differences (Figure 3). After completing six months of treatment, home practice with relaxation and propranolol were both tapered to discontinued. Headache resurgence was defined as an increase in headache activity of at least 50%. Return of headaches was significantly more frequent among patients treated with propranolol ($P<0.001$), demonstrating a superior long-term prophylactic effect with non-drug therapy. It is also likely that benefits from relaxation were retained since patients may have continued to use skills as needed after they discontinued regular daily practice.

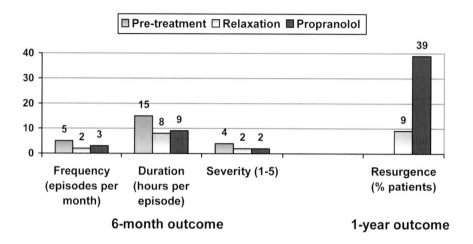

Figure 3 Six-month headache improvement with relaxation vs. propranolol. Headache severity was rated on a 5-point scale from 1 (mild) to 5 (severe). After six months, home practice with relaxation and propranolol were both tapered to discontinued. Headache resurgence was defined as an increase in headache activity of at least 50%. (Based on Kaushik 2005.)

Stress management

Stress is reported as a headache trigger by about three of every four patients with primary headaches. The occurrence of life stressors is linked to both headache frequency and severity [16]. Stress may also be an important factor in the development of new headache, with high work stress resulting in a 26% increased risk for developing new onset migraine [17].

Stress management is designed to improve headaches by altering the body's physiological response when encountering stress. Examples of helpful techniques include:

◆ autogenic training - changing the body's physiological response to stress;
◆ cognitive restructuring - changing one's thoughts about stress;
◆ distraction - minimizing focusing on stress.

For example, a student may develop a stress response before an exam - experiencing anxiety, a racing heart, tension in the neck and jaw muscles, and diarrhea. A stress management approach might include using deep breathing and relaxation techniques to reduce the physiological response. The student can also be trained to alter self messages from anxious and hopeless thoughts about the exam to positive thoughts ("I am well prepared for this test. I understand the material. I have performed well on previous tests. This exam will make up only part of my overall grade.") In the days prior to the exam, the student might be encouraged to fill study breaks with distracting physical activity, such as jogging or biking, rather than sitting around with friends worrying.

Stress management consisting of autogenic and cognitive therapies results in significantly decreased headache frequency and medication consumption in patients with migraine, a tension-type headache, or a mixed headache pattern [18]. Furthermore, a comparison of eight weeks of treatment with stress management versus amitriptyline (25-75mg daily) showed greater benefits with stress management (Figure 4) [19]. Although

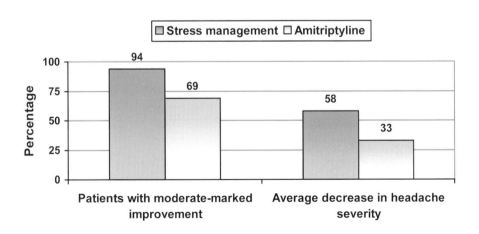

Figure 4 Comparison of stress management and amitriptyline. (Based on Cordingley 1990.)

higher doses of amitriptyline may have improved benefit in the medication-treated group, the stress management group showed good improvement in this study.

Butterbur

Butterbur (*Petasites hybridus*) is a perennial shrub. Butterbur root extract reduces inflammation and is used to treat asthma and migraine. Studies have consistently demonstrated good efficacy with butterbur. The number of migraine attacks decreased by 34-42% in patients treated with 50mg of butterbur root extract twice daily for three months [20, 21]. Furthermore, three months of treatment with 75mg butterbur extract twice daily decreased migraines by 58% [21]. Patients typically experience few side effects although about one in four will experience digestive system complaints, most commonly burping.

Moderately effective therapies

Moderately effective therapies are best used in conjunction with other, more effective treatments and are generally not used as monotherapy. Some patients will benefit from the addition of these techniques, although they are generally less effective than traditional medications, relaxation, stress management, and butterbur.

Diet

Putative headache triggers include foods that are rich in proteins known to affect vascular activity, such as tyramine (aged cheeses, alcohol, sour cream), phenylethylamine (chocolate), nitrates (hot dogs), and dopamine (broad bean pods). Suggested headache diets typically restrict foods rich in these compounds (Table 4). In general, these dietary restrictions are probably beneficial for only about one in three migraine sufferers and not beneficial for other chronically recurring headaches.

Table 4 Headache diet.

Food category	Specific foods to avoid
Beverages	Alcohol Caffeinated drinks (limit to 2 cups/day)
Breads and cereals	Donuts Fresh yeast breads
Dairy	Aged cheeses (blue, brie, camembert, emmenthal, gouda, gruyere, stilton) Buttermilk Sour cream Yogurt (limit to ½ cup per day)
Fruit	Bananas Citrus fruits Figs Kiwis Mangos Papaya Plums Raisins Strawberries
Meats	Aged or cured meat (bacon, bologna, pepperoni, salami, sausage) Peanuts and peanut butter Pickled herring Snails
Vegetables	Avocados Beans Corn Eggplant Olives Onions Pickles and pickled food Sauerkraut Spinach Snow peas Tomatoes and tomato products
Sweets	Chocolate
Food additives	Aspartame Meat tenderizer Monosodium glutamate

The effectiveness of dietary restrictions was evaluated in a study comparing headache activity in migraine sufferers assigned to one of three diets for 18 weeks: their usual diet, a structured diet restricting putative headache trigger foods, or a structured diet requiring high consumption of possible trigger foods [22]. Headache improved similarly when following either structured diet, with headache activity generally unrelated to specific food ingestion (Figure 5). Headaches, however, did seem to occur more frequently when patients had been fasting, drank alcohol, or ate chocolate. Citrus and nuts were also identified as possible aggravating food items. Widespread restrictions of foods containing tyramine, nitrates, and dopamine were not helpful, suggesting a limited role for dietary elimination in headache management.

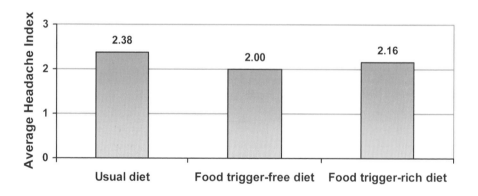

Figure 5 Effect of dietary restriction on headache. Headache severity was calculated using a headache index for which the sum of daily headache severity scores is divided by the number of days assessed. Headache severity was rated as 0=none, 1=mild, 2=moderate, and 3=severe. (Based on Diamond 1978.)

Two studies have evaluated headache relationship to individual food ingestion with either aspartame or chocolate. Large daily doses of aspartame for four weeks increased headache frequency but not severity in migraineurs who previously reported that aspartame was a headache trigger [23]. Study participants ingested very large doses of aspartame (300mg) four times a day, the equivalent of consuming 12 cans of diet soda or 32 packets of sweetener every day for a month. More moderate use was not tested; however, this study showed only a small increase in headache after regularly eating very large amounts of aspartame. A second study directly tested chocolate ingestion as a trigger in 63 women with chronic headaches by asking the women to follow a restrictive diet eliminating typical putative headache trigger foods and then consume 60g chocolate-flavored bars on four occasions, with headache activity measured before and after consumption [24]. Two of these bars were chocolate and two were carob, which does not contain putative trigger chemicals. All samples were flavored with mint to prevent identifying which bars were the actual chocolate bars. Even women who reported they believed chocolate triggered their headaches did not have headaches triggered with the blinded chocolate more often than with the carob placebo. Cheating on the diet and eating other restrictive foods like peanut butter, colas, or pizza (fresh yeast bread plus tomato sauce) along with chocolate did not increase headache activity.

While consuming specific foods is usually not linked to headache exacerbation, fasting has consistently been shown to aggravate headache and should be avoided by consuming regular meals and snacks throughout the day [25-27]. Furthermore, adequate hydration may also reduce headaches. In a small pilot study, increasing daily fluid intake by one liter daily resulted in modest reductions in headache activity [28].

Exercise and physical therapy

Musculoskeletal dysfunction can be identified in the majority of patients with primary headaches, with postural abnormalities and myofascial trigger points each affecting about eight in every ten headache patients [29]. Whether musculoskeletal changes represent a primary cause of head pain or a secondary consequence, therapy targeting muscles can help reduce contributory musculoskeletal abnormalities, as well as reduce pain by enhancing release of pain-relieving chemicals like endorphins. Aerobic exercise, targeted neck exercises, and oral appliances have demonstrated benefit for headache reduction.

Aerobic exercise showed benefit as headache prevention in a controlled study randomizing 20 migraineurs to standard aerobic exercise, three times per week for six weeks or a wait list control [30]. Pain severity decreased by 44% and pain duration by 36% in the exercise group, with no changes in headache activity in the control group. In a more recent study, 36 migraine patients were likewise instructed to perform aerobic exercise (10-minute warm-up, 20 minutes aerobics, 10-minute cool-down) three times per week for six weeks [31]. This open-label study reported similar reductions in headache frequency, severity, and duration (Figure 6).

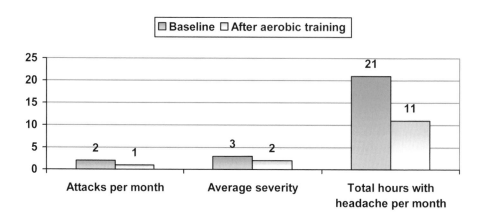

Figure 6 Effects of aerobic exercise. Headache severity was rated as 1=headache not requiring medication, 2=no disability after taking medication, 3=partial disability after medication, 4=total disability after medication. All changes from baseline were significant (P<0.0001). (Based on Köseoglu 2003.)

Stretching exercises of the neck may help reduce headache frequency, as well as acutely reduce pain during a headache episode. Performing stretching exercises in the shower or warm bath or first putting a heating pad on the neck for 15 minutes may assist in achieving a more complete and effective stretch. If pain persists after stretching, ice packs may help. A crossover treatment study compared headache reduction after treatment with physical therapy (including modalities and instructions in home stretching exercises) or relaxation with biofeedback [32]. Initial treatment with physical therapy was beneficial for only 14%, compared with 41% treated with relaxation. After crossing over to receive the alternative therapy, 47% who had failed to benefit with relaxation did experience significant headache reduction when physical therapy was added. Physical therapy may, therefore, be a useful adjunctive treatment for those who failed an initial course of more effective non-medication therapy.

Muscle contraction of craniomandibular muscles may also contribute to headache activity. Effective methods to reduce muscle tension include relaxation techniques, exercise, and intraoral splints. Intraoral appliances have demonstrated efficacy in patients with primary headache, like migraine [33]. The number of migraine attacks was reduced by 40% in 19 migraineurs treated with nocturnal occusal appliances [34]. The Nociceptive Trigeminal Inhibition (NTI) appliance is an FDA-approved migraine prevention treatment (www.nti-tss.com) in which an acrylic mini-splint fits over the incisors to reduce jaw clenching. In a randomized study, migraine patients with pericranial muscle tenderness were treated with either a full coverage occlusal splint or the NTI mini-splint [35]. All patients wore splints for two months at night and during times of stress. After eight weeks, migraine frequency decreased by 38% in the full occlusal splint group, similar to results from the earlier small study referenced above [34]. Migraineurs randomized to the NTI splint experienced significantly greater improvement, with a 62% decrease in migraine frequency ($P<0.05$). Oral devices, therefore, may be considered in patients with a primary headache associated with pericranial muscle tenderness.

Massage

Massage of the temples, head, and neck is often perceived as soothing during a headache attack. Although data are limited, modest benefit has been reported for massage therapy for migraine and tension-type headaches [36]. Therefore, while massage should not be used as monotherapy, it may provide adjunctive benefit.

Sleep regulation

Change in sleep is identified as a frequent headache trigger for one in every five patients with chronic headache [37, 38]. Both over- and under-sleeping are reported to aggravate chronic headaches (Figure 7) [38]. Therefore, patients with a chronic headache should be advised to sleep between six to eight hours each night. Table 5 describes strategies for achieving better sleep.

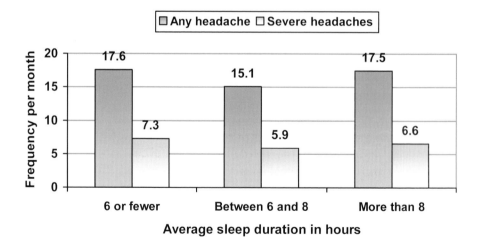

Figure 7 Effect of typical sleep duration on headache. Differences reached statistical significance for the insufficient sleep group (P<0.01). Differences were not statistically significant for the excessive sleep group, likely due to a relatively small number of patients in this sample (N=73). (Based on Kelman 2005.)

Table 5 Strategies for improving sleep.

- Plan to sleep more than 6 hours per night, but no more than 8 hours

- Use bed only for sleep and sex. Don't watch television in bed

- Establish and maintain regular sleep and rise times

- Avoid daytime naps if there are problems sleeping at night

- Avoid evening stimulants (caffeine, nicotine)

- Do aerobic exercise daily. Add 15 minutes of stretching before bed

- Practice relaxation techniques at bedtime

In an open-label study, taking 3mg of melatonin 30 minutes before bedtime for three months reduced migraine frequency by 61% and severity by 51% [39]. A few people taking melatonin reported side effects of excessive sleepiness, hair loss, and increased sexual libido. Controlled data are not available at this time.

Nicotine cessation

Consuming nicotine-containing products alters several important neurochemicals that influence headache activity, including endorphins [40], serotonin, norepinephrine, and dopamine [41]. The effect of nicotine on a variety of important neurotransmitters may help explain both reports of changes in stress perception and anxiety with smoking and the difficulty with smoking cessation. Smokers are more likely to develop chronic headaches compared with non-smokers. For example, the hazard ratio for incident migraine in smokers compared with people never smoking is 1.35 (95% CI: 1.08-1.68) [42]. Furthermore, headache frequency and severity are increased in heavier nicotine users [43]. Smoking cessation has been reported anecdotally to reduce headache activity; however, no controlled studies have been conducted in migraineurs. Nicotine discontinuation has been shown to be effective in reducing cluster headaches [44].

Nutritional supplements, vitamins, and herbs

A variety of nutritional therapies have been studied as headache-relieving therapies. Most nutritional therapies are used as prevention, while topical peppermint oil can provide acute headache relief. Each individual agent is described briefly below, with recommended effective doses provided in Table 6.

Table 6 Recommended doses of nutritional products for headache.

Acute therapy
- Topical peppermint oil: 10g peppermint oil in alcohol applied to forehead and temples during a headache

Prevention treatment
- Minerals and vitamins
  - Magnesium: 600mg daily
  - Riboflavin: 400mg daily
  - Coenzyme Q10: 150mg daily

- Herbs
  - Butterbur: 50-100mg twice daily
  - Feverfew: 100mg of feverfew containing 0.2% parthenolide daily

Acute treatment with topical peppermint oil

Peppermint oil is derived from the plant *Mentha piperita*, with the main active components menthol and menthon. Peppermint reduces gastric distress and acts as a topical analgesic. A solution of 10g peppermint oil in alcohol may be applied lightly to the forehead and temples during a headache attack and repeated after 15 and 30 minutes. In one study, topical peppermint oil reduced tension-type headache pain by 19% after 30 minutes and 34% after one hour [45]. Although not specifically tested for other headaches, topical peppermint oil may also be worth trying for acute migraines. Peppermint oil should never be applied to the faces of infants or small children, as this may result in glottal or bronchial spasm and respiratory distress.

Prevention treatment with minerals and vitamins

Daily adult requirements of magnesium for good health are about 300-400mg. This amount could be reached by eating two to three ounces of roasted pumpkin seeds or three to four bowls of bran cereal daily. Magnesium levels in the blood are often low in migraineurs. In one study, a 600mg magnesium supplement daily reduced the number of migraine attacks by 42% and severity by 34% [46]. The most common side effect with magnesium is diarrhea, which occurs in about one in five patients treated with magnesium.

The normal, daily recommended amount of riboflavin for general health in adults is 1-2mg. This amount would be found in about two cups of milk or yogurt. High dosed riboflavin (400mg of riboflavin daily for three months) reduced the number of migraine attacks by half, with no change in migraine severity [47, 48]. Furthermore, one study showed similar migraine prevention with either 400mg of riboflavin daily or standard migraine prevention medications [49].

Coenzyme Q10, also called ubiquinone and CoQ10, is made by the body and can also be obtained by eating meats and seafood. Coenzyme Q10 dosed 100mg three times daily or 150mg once daily for three months reduced migraine frequency by 27-55% [50, 51]. Improvement was better with the 150mg daily dose and both doses were well tolerated with very few side effects. Coenzyme Q10 can affect blood sugar metabolism and may change blood clotting, which may restrict use in patients with diabetes or bleeding disorders or using anticoagulants.

Prevention treatment with herbs

Feverfew (*Tanacetum parthenium L.*) comes from a flower that looks like a daisy. Its main active ingredient is parthenolide. Feverfew reduces inflammation and is commonly used to treat fevers, arthritis, menstrual discomfort, and migraines. Feverfew decreases migraines when people take 50-143mg of feverfew daily for three to four months [52]. With about 100mg of feverfew daily, migraine frequency decreases by 24% and migraine severity by 45%. Parthenolide content varies widely among different brands of feverfew. Feverfew must contain at least 0.2% parthenolide to prevent migraines [52]. A higher amount of parthenolide

(0.5%) is available in feverfew manufactured in Israel (at Galilee Herbal Remedies). This higher concentration may be more beneficial for reducing migraines. Feverfew decreases clotting and is restricted in patients with bleeding disorders or using aspirin, anti-inflammatory medications, or other medications that decrease clotting.

Ineffective therapies

Acupuncture can be a useful therapy for acute pain, such as dental pain. Acupuncture has been widely used to treat a variety of chronic pain conditions, although studies generally show no better efficacy than usual care treatment, placebo, or sham acupuncture [53]. Acupuncture has been extensively tested as a migraine preventive therapy. Studies consistently show no better result from patients randomized to receive real acupuncture versus sham acupuncture [54].

Botulinum toxin type A is routinely used in cosmetic procedures to reduce facial lines and has been tested in multiple trials as a migraine preventive agent. A recent review evaluating the published efficacy of migraine preventive therapies determined that the available evidence does not support recommending botulinum toxin injections as migraine prevention [54].

Conclusions

Effective non-medication and nutritional treatments, such as relaxation, stress management, and butterbur, may be used to complement traditional medications or as alternative monotherapy prevention. In general, benefits are maximized by combining medication and non-medication treatments. Therefore, patients may wish to use an effective acute therapy for their infrequent, severe migraines (such as a triptan) plus relaxation, stress management, aerobic exercise, and sleep regulation to help reduce headache frequency and severity. Non-medication techniques can also be combined with standard headache prevention medications. Utilizing a variety of non-medication techniques in conjunction with effective medications maximizes the likelihood of headache reduction.

Key Summary

◆ Effective non-traditional therapies for chronic headache include relaxation techniques, stress management, and butterbur.

◆ Effective non-medication therapies offer a similar benefit to standard headache prevention medications and may be used as first-line or monotherapy.

◆ Moderately effective complementary therapies include exercise, lifestyle changes, and some nutritional products.

◆ Moderately effective treatments may complement more effective non-medication or medication treatments.

◆ A lack of a convincing effect for reducing chronic headache has consistently been demonstrated for acupuncture and botulinum toxin injections.

References

1. Niskar AS, Peled-Leviatan T, Garty-Sandalon N. Who uses complementary and alternative medicine in Israel? *J Altern Complement Med* 2007; 13: 989-995.

2. Lim MK, Sadarangani P, Chan HL, Heng JY. Complementary and alternative medicine use in multiracial Singapore. *Complement Ther Med* 2005; 13: 16-24.

3. Rössler W, Lauber C, Angst J, *et al.* The use of complementary and alternative medicine in the general population: results from a longitudinal community study. *Psychol Med* 2007; 37: 73-84.

4. Tindle HA, Davis RB, Phillips RS, Eisenberg DM. Trends in use of complementary and alternative medicine by US adults: 1997-2002. *Altern Ther Health Med* 2005; 11: 42-49.

5. Thomas K, Coleman P. Use of complementary or alternative medicine in a general population in Great Britain. Results from the National Omnibus survey. *J Public Health* (Oxf) 2004; 26: 152-157.

6. Hammond DC. Review of the efficacy of clinical hypnosis with headaches and migraines. *Int J Clin Exp Hypn* 2007; 55: 207-219.

7. Ben-Arye E, Frenkel M, Klein A, Scharf M. Attitudes toward integration of complementary and alternative medicine in primary care: perspectives of patients, physicians and complementary practitioners. *Patient Educ Couns* 2008; 70: 395-402.

8. Holroyd KA, France JL, Cordingley GE, *et al*. Enhancing the effectiveness of relaxation-thermal biofeedback training with propranolol hydrochloride. *J Consult Clin Psychol* 1995; 63: 327-330.

9. Nuti A, Lucetti C, Pavaese N, *et al*. Long-term follow-up after flunarizine or nimodipine discontinuation in migraine patients. *Cephalalgia* 1996; 16: 337-340.

10. Kaniecki R. Long-term results of interval prophylaxis of migraine: a prospective, randomized, controlled clinical trial. *Headache* 1997; 37: 315.

11. Rothrock JF, Mendizabal JE. An analysis of the 'carry-over effect' following successful short-term treatment of transformed migraine with divalproex sodium. *Headache* 2000; 40: 17-19.

12. Diener H, Agosti R, Allais G, *et al*. Cessation versus continuation of 6-month migraine preventive therapy with topiramate (PROMPT): a randomized, double-blind, placebo-controlled trial. *Lancet Neurol* 2007; 6: 1054-1062.

13. Warner G, Lance JW. Relaxation therapy in migraine and chronic tension headache. *Med J Australia* 1975; 1: 298-301.

14. Daly EJ, Donn PA, Galliher MJ, Zimmerman JS. Biofeedback applications to migraine and tension headache: a double-blinded outcome study. *Biofeedback & Self-Regulation* 1983; 8: 135-152.

15. Kaushik R, Kaushik RM, Mahajan SK, Rajesh V. Biofeedback-assisted diaphragmatic breathing and systematic relaxation versus propranolol in long-term prophylaxis of migraine. *Complement Ther Med* 2005; 13: 165-174.

16. Fernandez E, Sheffield J. Relative contributions of life events versus daily hassles to the frequency and intensity of headache. *Headache* 1996; 36: 595-602.

17. Mäki K, Vahtera J, Virtanen M, *et al*. Work stress and new-onset migraine in a female employee population. *Cephalalgia* 2008;28:18-25.

18. Zsombok T, Juhasz G, Budavari A, Vitrai J, Bagdy G. Effect of autogenic training on drug consumption in patients with primary headache: an 8-month follow-up study. *Headache* 2003; 43: 251-257.

19. Cordingley G, Holrody K, Pingel J, Jerome A, Nash J. Amitriptyline versus stress management therapy in the prophylaxis of chronic tension headache. *Headache* 1990; 30: 300.

20. Diener HC, Rahlfs VW, Danesch U. The first placebo-controlled trial of a special butterbur root extract for the prevention of migraine: reanalysis of efficacy criteria. *Eur Neurol* 2004; 51: 89-97.

21. Lipton RB, Göbel H, Einhäupl KM, Wilks K, Mauskop A. *Petasites hybridus* root (butter bur) is an effective preventive treatment for migraine. *Neurology* 2004; 63: 2240-2244.

22. Medina JC, Diamond S. The role of diet in migraine. *Headache* 1978; 18: 31-34.

23. Koehler SM, Glaros A. The effect of aspartame on migraine headache. *Headache* 1988; 28: 10-14.

24. Marcus DA, Scharff L, Turk DC, Gourley LM. A double-blind provocative study of chocolate as a trigger for headache. *Cephalalgia* 997; 17: 855-862.

25. Medina JL, Diamond S. The role of diet in migraine. *Headache* 1978; 18: 31-34.

26. Mosek A, Korczyn AD. Yom Kippur headache. *Neurology* 1995; 45: 1953-1955.

27. Topacoglu H, Karcioglu O, Yuruktumen A, *et al.* Impact of Ramadan on demographics and frequencies of disease-related visits in the emergency department. *Int J Clin Pract* 2005; 59: 900-905.

28. Spigt MG, Kuijper EC, Schayck CP, *et al.* Increasing daily water intake for prophylactic treatment of headache: a pilot trial. *Eur J Neurol* 2005; 12: 715-718.

29. Marcus DA, Scharff L, Mercer SR, Turk DC. Musculoskeletal abnormalities in chronic headache: a controlled comparison of headache diagnostic groups. *Headache* 1999; 39: 21-27.

30. Lockett DC, Campbell JF. The effects of aerobic exercise on migraine. *Headache* 1992; 32: 50-54.

31. Köseoglu E, Akboyraz A, Soyuer A, Ersoy AO. Aerobic exercise and plasma beta endorphin levels in patients with migrainous headache without aura. *Cephalalgia* 2003; 23: 972-976.

32. Marcus DA, Scharff L, Mercer SR, Turk DC. Nonpharmacological treatment for migraine: incremental utility of physical therapy with relaxation and thermal biofeedback. *Cephalalgia* 1998; 18: 266-272.

33. Shevel E. Craniomandibular muscles, intraoral orthoses and migraine. *Expert Rev Neurothrapeutics* 2005; 5: 371-377.

34. Lamey PJ, Steele JG, Aitchison T. Migraine: the effect of acrylic appliance design on clinical response. *Br Dent J* 1996; 180: 137-140.

35. Shankland WE. Migraine and tension-type headache reduction through pericranial muscular suppression: a preliminary report. *Cranio* 2001; 19: 269-278.

36. Tsao JI. Effectiveness of massage therapy for chronic, non-malignant pain: a review. *Evid Based Complement Alternat Med* 2007; 4: 165-179.

37. Marcus DA. Chronic headache: the importance of trigger identification. *Headache & Pain* 2003; 14: 139-144.

38. Kelman L, Rains JC. Headache and sleep: examination of sleep patterns and complaints in a large clinical sample of migraineurs. *Headache* 2005; 45: 904-910.

39. Peres MP, Zukerman E, da Cunha Tanuri F, Moreira FR, Cipolla-Neto J. Melatonin, 3mg, is effective for migraine prevention. *Neurology* 2004; 63: 757.

40. Pomerleau OF. Endogenous opioids and smoking - a review of progress and problems. *Psychoneuroendocrinology* 1998; 23: 115-130.

41. Mansbach RS, Rovetti CC, Freeland CS. The role of monoamine neurotransmitters system in the nicotine discriminative stimulus. *Drug Alcohol Depend* 1998; 23: 115-130.

42. Hozawa A, Houston T, Steffes MW, *et al.* The association of cigarette smoking with self-reported disease before middle age: the Coronary Artery Risk Development in Young Adults (CARDIA) study. *Prev Med* 2006; 42: 193-199.

43. Payne TJ, Stetson B, Stevens VM, Johnson CA, Penzien DB, Van Dorsten B. Impact of cigarette smoking on headache activity in headache patients. *Headache* 1991; 31: 329-332.

44. Millac P, Akhtar N. Cigarette smoking and cluster headache. *Headache* 1985; 25: 220.
45. Göbel H, Fresenius J, Heinze A, Dworschak M, Soyka D. Effectiveness of *Oleum menthae piperitae* and paracetamol in therapy of headache of the tension type. *Nervenarzt* 1996; 67: 672-681.
46. Peikert A, Wilimzig C, Köhne-Volland R. Prophylaxis of migraine with oral magnesium: results from a prospective, multicenter, placebo-controlled and double-blind randomized study. *Cephalalgia* 1996; 16: 257-263.
47. Schoenen J, Jacquy J, Lenaerts M. Effectiveness of high-dose riboflavin in migraine prophylaxis: a randomized controlled trial. *Neurology* 1998; 50: 466-470.
48. Boehnke C, Reuter U, Flach U, *et al.* High-dose riboflavin treatment is efficacious in migraine prophylaxis: an open study in a tertiary care center. *Eur J Neurol* 2004; 11: 475-477.
49. Sándor PS, Áfra J, Ambrosini A, Schoenen J. Prophylactic treatment of migraine with ß-blockers and riboflavin: differential effects on the intensity dependence of auditory evoked cortical potentials. *Headache* 2000; 40: 30-35.
50. Rozen TD, Oshinsky ML, Geneline CA, *et al.* Open label trial of coenzyme Q10 as a migraine preventive. *Cephalalgia* 2002; 22: 137-141.
51. Sándor PS, Di Clemente L, Coppola G, *et al.* Efficacy of coenzyme Q10 in migraine prophylaxis: a randomized controlled trial. *Neurology* 2005; 64: 713-715.
52. Rios J, Passe MM. Evidence-based use of botanicals, minerals, and vitamins in the prophylactic treatment of migraine. *J Am Acad Nurs Pract* 2004; 16: 251-256.
53. Ezzo J, Berman B, Hadhazy VA, *et al.* Is acupuncture effective for the treatment of chronic pain? A systematic review. *Pain* 2000; 86: 217-225.
54. Schürks M, Diener H, Goadsby P. Update on the prophylaxis of migraine. *Curr Treat Opt Neurol* 2008; 10: 20-29.

Chapter 8
Managing headaches in children and women

Children and adolescents

The same treatments used for adult headache are often effective in pediatric patients, although dosage adjustment is necessary. The European Federation of Neurological Sciences (EFNS) task force has provided guidelines for effective migraine treatment in children and adolescents (Table 1) [1]. These same recommendations were echoed in a subsequent report by the European Headache Federation [2].

Table 1 Effective migraine treatments in children and adolescents (Based on Evers 2006.)

Treatment	Dosage
Acute treatment Ibuprofen	10mg/kg
Acetaminophen/paracetamol	15mg/kg
Domperidone (for nausea)	10mg (not available in Canada and the United States)
Sumatriptan nasal spray	10mg after age 12
Zolmitriptan	2.5-5mg after age 12
Prevention Flunarizine	10mg daily
Propranolol	40-80mg daily

Acute treatment

Subsequent to the EFNS report recommendations (Table 1), two studies were published demonstrating good efficacy of oral rizatriptan (5mg for children weighing 20-39kg and 10mg for children ≥40kg) in children and adolescents from ages 6-17 and zolmitriptan nasal spray in adolescents 12-17 years old [3, 4]. A summary of headache relief (reduction from severe to mild or none) with triptans in placebo-controlled studies is shown in Figure 1 [3-6]. All studies included adolescents ≥12 years old, with children six and older included only in the oral zolmitriptan and rizatriptan studies. Ibuprofen was dosed 200mg in children under 12 and 400mg for adolescents in the oral zolmitriptan study [6].

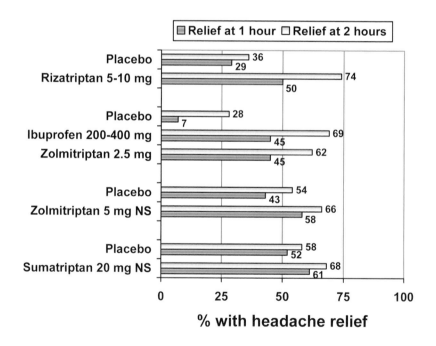

Figure 1 Efficacy of triptans in children and adolescents. NS=nasal spray. Triptan response superior to placebo (P<0.05) was as follows: sumatriptan NS at 2 hours, zolmitriptan NS at 1 hour, zolmitriptan and ibuprofen each at 1 and 2 hours, and rizatriptan at 1 and 2 hours. (Based on Ahonen 2006, Lewis 2007, Winner 2006, Evers/Rahmann 2006.)

Prevention

Good efficacy for prevention has been demonstrated with propranolol and flunarizine [6]. Antidepressants and anti-epileptics have also demonstrated efficacy in pediatric headache patients [7-10]. Controlled trials have not evaluated selective serotonin reuptake inhibitors (SSRIs) for pediatric migraine prevention, although their efficacy is relatively low in adult headache. SSRIs have been linked to a small but significantly increased risk of suicidal ideation/attempt in pediatric patients treating mood disorders [11]. Consequently, careful monitoring is required when using SSRIs.

Complementary and alternative treatments

Relaxation, stress management, and biofeedback are effective non-pharmacological headache therapies in pediatric patients [12, 13]. Healthy lifestyle habits, including daily exercise, balanced meals, and adequate sleep, should be promoted. Sleep disturbances, including insufficient total sleep, occur in the majority of pediatric headache patients, especially those with migraine [14, 15]. Scheduling should require regular times for retiring to bed with lights off and rising in the morning. Children and adolescents should not be permitted to watch television after bedtime.

Few vitamins, minerals, and herbs have been tested in pediatrics. One large study treated children and adolescents with migraine with magnesium for four months [16]. Magnesium dosage varied according to weight. Magnesium decreased the number of days with migraine by 45%. Migraines were also less severe with magnesium. Tension-type headaches in children and adolescents may also be substantially reduced with magnesium [17]. Butterbur root extract was likewise tested in children and adolescents with migraine [18]. Taking 25-75mg (depending on their weight) of butterbur extract twice daily for four months decreased the number of migraines by 63%. Both children and adolescents experienced a similar degree of migraine relief with butterbur. As in adults, the most common side effect was burping.

Recalcitrant headache treatment

In some cases, headaches result in significant disability in children and adolescents, typically manifest by school absence. Treatment begins with resuming a regular routine, with good school participation the top priority [19]. In most circumstances, attending school will not aggravate the pain complaints and will serve as a distraction from pain and the sick role. Prolonged school absence results in isolation and fear of both academic and social deficiencies, additional stressors that may further aggravate headache complaints. The social and emotional development advantages of attending school cannot be duplicated with a homebound education environment. The longer school absence is maintained, the more difficult it is for children to return to school because of failure to maintain academic work and fear of isolation from peers on return to school.

Children experiencing repeated school absence due to headache should:

◆ receive a complete evaluation to verify headache diagnosis;
◆ be prescribed effective medication and non-medication treatments;
◆ receive specialized training in relaxation, cognitive behavioral therapy techniques, and distraction from a psychologist skilled in teaching pain management techniques;
◆ have a regular home routine initiated, including regular bed times (with no television after bed time) and regular meal times (including breakfast);
◆ schedule daily aerobic exercise;
◆ have instructions given to the parents that the child should go to school even on days with a headache unless she is vomiting. She will then need to be taken to school after vomiting ceases;
◆ have instructions given to the school nurse that the child may stay in the nurse's office for up to one hour with a headache and then return to class.

Family therapy will be necessary when parents are hesitant to insist on school attendance to help parents develop strategies for ensuring school participation, as well as identification of manipulative behaviors that erode parents' resolve to encourage activity normalization. Remind parents that childhood migraine attacks typically last only one to two hours, so missing an entire day of school is not reasonable.

Women

Managing headaches affected by changes in reproductive status in women focuses on either minimizing changes in estradiol levels with estrogen supplementation when a decline in estradiol levels is expected to aggravate chronic headaches (e.g., with menses) or by manipulating other important neurochemicals, such as using antidepressants or triptans to modulate serotonin levels, valproate or gabapentin to modulate gamma-aminobutyric acid, or antinausea medications to modulate dopamine [20]. Treatment effects on the developing fetus must also be considered in women of childbearing potential to ensure safe treatments during attempted conception, pregnancy, and lactation.

Oral contraceptives

Headache aggravation with oral contraceptives (OCPs) is usually experienced as a clustering of headaches when estradiol levels drop during the first few days of the placebo week of cycling OCPs. Headache aggravation has been reported in 18-50% of migraineurs using OCPs [21-23]. Discontinuation of OCPs reduces headache for most women; however, improvement may be delayed for up to one year.

Headache associated with OCPs may be managed by reducing peak-to-trough changes in estrogen by:

◆ reducing estrogen dose;
◆ supplementing low dose estrogen during the placebo week;
◆ reducing the duration of the placebo week, including eliminating the placebo week from most cycles.

Women experiencing exacerbations in headache with OCPs may need alternative contraception. A significant change in migraine characteristics after using OCPs should result in a prompt change to alternative contraception rather than adjustment of estradiol dosage. If aura symptoms worsen or new aura symptoms develop after beginning OCPs, OCPs should be discontinued and alternative contraception started because of a small, but significant increased stroke risk in migraineurs with aura [24].

Menstrual headache

Menstrually-linked headaches may be treated by implementing hormonal therapy or mini-prophylaxis with standard headache medications (Table 2). Interestingly, although short-term prevention medications typically do not improve non-menstrual headache, either a short course of a new preventive or a temporary dosage increase in maintenance prevention therapy perimenstrually often reduces menstrually-triggered headaches.

Table 2 Treatment of menstrual headache.

Perimenstrual hormone therapy
- 7-day 100mg estrogen patch

- Eliminate placebo week from oral contraceptives for 2 or 3 months

Mini-prophylaxis with standard headache therapies
- Usual dosage should be taken for 3 days before the expected menstrual period and during first 2-4 days of menses

- Standard acute headache medications
    - Non-steroidal anti-inflammatory drugs
    - 2.5mg naratriptan twice daily
    - 2.5mg frovatriptan once or twice daily

- Standard headache preventive medications
    - ß-blocker
    - Antidepressants
    - Calcium channel blocker
    - Neurostabilizing anti-epileptics

Pregnancy and breastfeeding

While most chronic headaches experienced during pregnancy are usually primary headaches, important secondary headaches during pregnancy and postpartum include: low pressure headaches related to spinal anesthesia, eclampsia/pre-eclampsia, cerebral venous thrombosis, subarachnoid hemorrhage, intracranial tumors, idiopathic intracranial hypertension (pseudotumor cerebri), and meningitis (Table 3). Acute strokes, cerebral venous thrombosis, symptomatic brain tumors, and benign intracranial hypertension (pseudotumor cerebri) occur with increased frequency during pregnancy [25]. Pregnancy is also associated with an increased risk of subarachnoid hemorrhage, typically from ruptured arteriovenous malformations and postpartum cerebral venous thrombosis [25]. Cerebral venous thrombosis occurs in 10-20 women/100,000 deliveries, with nearly 80% of cases occurring during the first two postpartum weeks [26-28]. While tumor incidence does not increase with pregnancy, the growth of pituitary adenomas and meningiomas is accelerated during pregnancy [29, 30]. Benign intracranial hypertension (pseudotumor cerebri) may also be triggered by elevated estrogen, and may occur or worsen during pregnancy [31-33].

Table 3 Secondary headaches more common during or aggravated by pregnancy.

- Arteriovenous malformations

- Benign intracranial hypertension (pseudotumor cerebri)

- Brain tumors (e.g., pituitary adenomas and meningiomas)

- Central venous thrombosis

- Eclampsia

- Stroke (hemorrhagic and thrombotic)

Neuroimaging during pregnancy and lactation

In general, neuroimaging studies are not recommended for patients with chronic headache unless a new headache pattern develops or abnormal neurological signs or symptoms occur, such as focal abnormalities, mental status changes, or seizures [34]. Magnetic resonance imaging (MRI) is preferred over traditional radiographic testing during pregnancy. MRI exposure during pregnancy is generally considered to be safe [35], with no negative sequelae identified during evaluations of three-year-olds exposed to MRI *in utero* [36] or the offspring of female MRI technicians [37]. The American College of Radiology recommends MRI during pregnancy to avoid exposure to ionizing radiation when imaging studies are needed and the results of testing may change patient care [38]. Computed tomography (CT) may be needed in those cases where intracranial hemorrhage is suspected. Fetal exposure to ionizing radiation from a maternal head CT is extremely low (<0.005 mGy) and considered to be substantially less risky for the fetus than not identifying and treating potentially serious neurological conditions in the mother [39]. Furthermore, contrast agents may also be used, if indicated, during pregnancy and lactation. The 11th European Symposium on Urogenital Radiology conducted an extensive literature review of maternal iodinated and gadolinium contrast exposures during pregnancy and lactation [40]. Intra-uterine exposure to maternal iodinated contrast agents can depress fetal and neonatal thyroid function, necessitating screening for hypothyroidism during the infant's first week of life. There are no fetal effects from intra-uterine gadolinium exposure. Only small amounts of iodinated or gadolinium contrast agents are expected in breast milk. Consequently, temporary cessation of breastfeeding is unnecessary when contrast agents are used in lactating women [40].

Determining drug safety during pregnancy

The most widely used tool for evaluating drug safety during pregnancy in the United States is the Food and Drug Administration (FDA) safety rating system. Drugs listed as FDA risk categories A and B are considered to be relatively safe during pregnancy, C drugs may be used if benefits outweigh possible risks, and D and X drugs are generally avoided. A survey of FDA pregnancy risk category assignment of drugs in the 2001 and 2002 Physicians' Desk References revealed that >60% of drugs assigned a pregnancy risk category were risk category C [41]. Another risk categorizing system is the Teratogen Information System (TERIS), which catalogs risk of teratogenic effects for the offspring of exposed women as none, minimal, small, moderate, or high. When no or limited human data are available, a drug is classified as having an undetermined risk in the TERIS system. An unlikely rating is given when risk is considered to probably be very low; however, supportive data are limited.

Unfortunately, drugs are not necessarily assigned to comparable risk categories when comparing rating systems [42]. For example, pregnancy risk category assignment was compared for drugs common to three different classification systems: the United States FDA, the Australian Drug Evaluation Committee (ADEC), and the Swedish Catalogue of Approved Drugs (FASS) [43]. Only one in four of the drugs common to all three systems received the same risk factor category. Differences were attributed to disparity in definitions among the three systems, as well as dissimilarities in the way accessible literature was used to determine risk category.

Despite limitations with current safety rating systems, general recommendations can be made using the available literature to determine which medications are relatively safe to use during pregnancy and lactation. When treating headache during pregnancy and breastfeeding it is important to limit excessive use of over-the-counter pain remedies, dehydration, and pain-related disability. Generally accepted treatment recommendations are provided below.

Preconception counseling

The most serious medication effects on the fetus occur with early exposure, before many women are aware that they are pregnant. Therefore, management of young women with chronic headache needs to include an evaluation of reproductive status and contraceptive use. Fertile women not using effective contraception and at risk of pregnancy should be treated with those medications deemed safe during early pregnancy.

Smoking cessation is an important recommendation before and during pregnancy and also after delivery for the health of both mother and baby.

Cigarette use has been clearly linked to headache activity during pregnancy. A longitudinal survey of almost 5000 women experiencing a pregnancy over a 3.5-year period reported severe headache significantly more often in smokers compared with non-smokers (22% vs. 17%, P<0.001) [44].

Safe and effective headache treatments during pregnancy and lactation

Healthy lifestyle changes (e.g., like eating regular meals, achieving adequate sleep, and avoiding nicotine), aerobic exercise and physical therapy, and psychological pain management skills (e.g., relaxation techniques and stress management) are generally effective strategies to help minimize chronic primary headaches during pregnancy and lactation. A controlled clinical trial demonstrated both short- and long-term efficacy from relaxation with thermal biofeedback during pregnancy [45, 46]. Significant headache reduction occurred for 73% treated with biofeedback versus 29% assigned to an attention control [45]. Benefits were maintained up to one year postpartum in 68% of treated subjects [46]. Dietary restrictions are usually not helpful and are not recommended as they restrict important nutrients.

Medications during pregnancy

Informing patients about safe and effective headache therapies during pregnancy is important, even in women who report a preference to avoid medication exposure. One in every three women self-medicate for health symptoms during pregnancy, especially with analgesics [47-49]. Unsupervised use of analgesics can result in analgesic overuse headaches, as well as both maternal and fetal side effects. Acute headache therapies during pregnancy are typically restricted to analgesics and anti-emetics, providing good efficacy for headache management and safety for the baby. Preventive medications are more restricted. Safe treatments during pregnancy are provided in Table 4.

Table 4 Headache medication recommendations during pregnancy.

Safety rating	Acute treatment	Prevention
Relatively safe	Acetaminophen/paracetamol Caffeine Non-steroidal anti-inflammatory drugs during 2nd trimester Prednisone Topical peppermint oil Vitamin B6 or ginger for nausea	Magnesium
Use if benefits>risks	Aspirin Butalbital Dexamethasone Opioids Prochlorperazine Promethazine Triptans	Bupropion Flunarizine Gabapentin Lamotrigine Propranolol Timolol Topiramate Tricyclic antidepressants Venlafaxine
Avoid	Ergotamine Isometheptene	Atenolol Paroxetine Valproic acid

Early NSAID exposure during pregnancy has been linked to an increased risk of miscarriage. A post-hoc analysis of retrospectively collected data reported an 80% increased risk of miscarriage among NSAID users, with the risk highest when NSAIDs were used around the time of conception [50]. In this same report, paracetamol use was not linked to an increased miscarriage risk. While NSAIDs are generally restricted only during the third trimester in the United States due to significant effects on the ductus arteriosus, uterine contractions, or bleeding, their use is limited to the second trimester in many European countries. Recent recommendations from the EFNS based on review of scientific data from clinical trials and expert consensus opinion advised use of acetaminophen/paracetamol throughout pregnancy, with NSAIDs restricted to the second trimester [6].

Triptan safety has been evaluated during pregnancy through patient databases and voluntary registries. The most extensive data are available for sumatriptan. A national database review from Sweden (N=658 sumatriptan users) reported small, but not statistically significant increased risks for preterm and low-birth-weight babies when mothers used sumatriptan [51]. Data did not permit analysis of confounding factors, such as disease severity in sumatriptan users, which might have also influenced outcome. Due to the relatively small number of identified women who have used triptans during pregnancy, safety recommendations cannot be made at this time.

Recommendations from the American College of Obstetricians and Gynecologists include utilization of herbal and vitamin supplements for nausea, including vitamin B6 and ginger [52]. Opioids have limited efficacy in migraine and are generally reserved as rescue therapy. Prednisone may be used as rescue therapy when acute treatment has failed and disabling migraine is prolonged and unremitting.

Among headache preventive medications, beta-blockers have the best record for a combination of good efficacy and safety in pregnant women. Beta-blocker exposure may, however, increase the risk of neonatal hypoglycemia, hypotension, bradycardia, and respiratory depression. Atenolol exposure at conception or during the first trimester has been linked to low birth weight [53]. Older studies have similarly suggested a possible association between propranolol and intra-uterine growth retardation. Ideally, beta-blockers should be tapered within the last few weeks of pregnancy (starting around week 36) to minimize the effects on labor and the newborn baby. While calcium channel blockers were not linked to an increased risk of malformations in a large, Hungarian surveillance survey, experience in pregnancy is inadequate to recommend routine use for headache prevention during pregnancy [54].

Antidepressants have recently been linked to increased rates of spontaneous abortion in women using antidepressants compared with non-depressed women (12% vs. 4%, relative risk=1.45) [55]. No differences were found among antidepressant classes. Although these data do not determine whether the increased miscarriage rate was due to depression-related factors versus medication use, antidepressants should probably be selected as second-line preventive therapy after beta-blockers in pregnant women. Exposure to the selective serotonin reuptake inhibitor, paroxetine, during the first trimester has been associated with an increased risk of major malformations (odds ratio=2.2) and major cardiac malformations (odds ratio=3.1) among women using a daily dosage >25mg [56]. A recent report of pregnancy registry data identified a higher than expected incidence of cardiac abnormalities in babies exposed to bupropion *in utero* [57]. Furthermore, a small, prospective study comparing pregnancy outcome in 136 women using bupropion at least during their first trimester and 133 controls reported a significantly higher rate of spontaneous abortion (15% vs. 4%, P=0.009) in bupropion-exposed women [58].

Valproic acid is contraindicated during conception and pregnancy, due to teratogenic effects with neural tube defects. Gabapentin may be used in early pregnancy, but is typically discontinued in the third trimester because of possible interference with bony development. Small studies in epileptic women have not identified fetal effects with gabapentin treatment [59]. The Gabapentin Pregnancy Registry published data on 44 live births, with no increased risk of abortion, low birth weight, or malformation seen in gabapentin-exposed babies [59]. The very small number in this sample, however, substantially limits safety interpretations that can be made using these data. Early malformation report data suggest restricting topiramate use as a migraine preventive during pregnancy. Post-marketing data reported topiramate use in male babies with hypospadias [60]. A case report recently described the occurrence of limb and oral malformations after maternal treatment for epilepsy during pregnancy with topiramate [61].

Medications during lactation
Immediately following delivery, milk production is quite low for the first one to two postpartum days and medications given at this time are unlikely to be present in sufficient amounts to affect the newborn. After the first few days when milk production increases, concerns about mother-to-infant transfer of medications become more significant. Drug exposure to the nursing baby can be minimized by administering medications immediately after completing breastfeeding, allowing the ingested drug to be metabolized and excreted before the next breastfeeding session. If non-compatible drugs are used between feedings, breast milk might be

expressed and discarded for several hours after dosing, supplementing feeds with stored milk.

Both the American Academy of Pediatrics and the World Health Organization have offered guidelines for safe maternal medication exposures when breastfeeding [62, 63]. Table 5 details acute and prevention medication recommendations. Drug safety may depend on the age of the nursing baby, with the capacity to absorb and eliminate drugs different in premature infants and newborns in comparison with older babies. In general, extra caution should be exercised when administering drugs to nursing mothers of premature babies or infants <1 month old.

Table 5 Headache medication recommendations during lactation. (Based on American Academy Pediatrics 2001, WHO website.)

Safety rating	Acute treatment	Prevention
Compatible with nursing	Acetaminophen/paracetamol Ibuprofen Prednisone Sumatriptan	Magnesium Propranolol Riboflavin Timolol Valproic acid (if using adequate contraception) Verapamil
Compatible with nursing, but use caution monitoring baby for possible side effects	Aspirin Butorphanol Caffeine Naproxen Ondansetron Opioids Topical peppermint oil (avoid near baby's face)	Antidepressants Atenolol Lamotrigine
Avoid	Ergotamine Metoclopramide Promethazine	Flunarizine

Recommended acute headache medications with nursing include analgesics and sumatriptan [62]. Drug exposure to the nursing baby can be minimized by administering medications immediately after completing breastfeeding, allowing the ingested drug to be metabolized and excreted before the next breastfeeding session.

Some antihypertensives and valproate are compatible with breastfeeding [62]. Maternal antidepressants have generally not been linked to specific effects in the baby, with the exception of fluoxetine, which can cause colic, irritability, feeding and sleep disorders, and slow weight gain. Antidepressants, however, are of potential concern since they are excreted in breast milk and effects on the developing nervous system are unknown. Recently, the use of serotonin reuptake inhibitors, including SSRIs and serotonin and norepinephrine reuptake inhibitors, in the third trimester have been linked to a neonatal behavioral syndrome [64]. In comparison to babies with no *in utero* exposure to serotonin reuptake inhibitors or exposure during early pregnancy, babies exposed in the third trimester carry a risk ratio of 3.0 for the development of neonatal behavioral syndrome. Most cases have been reported with fluoxetine and paroxetine. Features typically include tremors/jitteriness, increased muscle tone/reflexes, feeding/digestive disturbances, irritability/agitation, respiratory disturbances, excessive crying, and sleep disturbances. In most cases, symptoms are mild and respond to supportive measures.

Menopause

Menopause is frequently associated with changing headache. The perimenopausal period when women are also experiencing other somatic symptoms, such as hot flashes, is a common time of headache exacerbation. Postmenopausally, headache is expected to improve because of the lack of cyclical estrogen changes. Migraine improves in 67% of migraineurs following spontaneous menopause, while worsening in 67% after surgical menopause [65]. Greater improvement with spontaneous menopause may be related to age, which decreases headache activity for both men and women [66, 67]. A significant change in headache pattern at any time should prompt a careful history and physical examination, followed by consideration of the need for additional testing. Although headache often increases in frequency and severity during the early perimenopausal period, a significant change in the quality or characteristics of the headache should prompt a more detailed evaluation.

Treatment of early menopausal symptoms with hormone replacement therapy (HRT) may result in alterations in headache, with an equal number of women reporting worsening or improvement of headache [68]. A prospective, longitudinal study compared headache activity before and after different HRT formulations in 54 women after spontaneous menopause [69]. Continuous, transdermal estradiol was least likely to aggravate migraine. Recommendations for treating headaches exacerbated by menopause or HRT are provided in Table 6.

Table 6 Treating headache during menopause.

- Determine if there has been a change in headache pattern notable enough to warrant additional evaluation

- Adjust HRT if it aggravates headache
    - Use non-cycling, transdermal route if able
    - Reduce estrogen dose
    - Change estrogen-replacement product

- Add standard headache-preventive therapy in conjunction with estrogen replacement

Conclusions

Headaches occurring in children, adolescents, and women at various stages of their reproductive cycles can be managed using the same principles that govern general headache treatment; however, medication selection and dosages used will often differ from standard adult headache therapy. Headache treatment in children and adolescents focuses on limiting disability by achieving good school attendance. Hormonally-triggered headaches in women may be improved through hormonal therapy or standard headache treatments. Headaches during pregnancy can be treated with effective non-medication treatments and selected medications. Menopausal headache exacerbations may be improved through adjusting hormone replacement therapy.

Key Summary

◆ Efficacy has been demonstrated for analgesics and some triptans in pediatric patients. Domperidone may be used adjunctively to treat headache-related nausea.

◆ Frequent headaches in children and adolescents may be effectively treated with relaxation, stress management, lifestyle modifications, flunarizine, propranolol, and butterbur.

◆ Headaches related to oral contraceptives or menstruation may be treated with hormonal therapy.

◆ Neuroimaging may be safely performed when necessary during pregnancy and lactation.

◆ Safe treatments during pregnancy include acute management with some analgesics and topical peppermint oil and prevention with relaxation, stress management, and magnesium. Propranolol also has a long track record of safe use during pregnancy, although risk classification recommends using only when benefits outweigh risks.

◆ Headache aggravation is common during the perimenopause, although a significant change in headache pattern should result in a careful evaluation for possible secondary headaches. Migraine later improves for two in every three women after completing spontaneous menopause.

References

1. Evers A, Áfra J, Frese A, *et al*. EFNS guideline on the drug treatment of migraine - report of an EFNS task force. *Eur J Neurol* 2006; 13: 560-572.

2. Steiner TJ, Paemeleire K, Jensen R, *et al*. European principles of management of common headache disorders in primary care. *J Headache Pain* 2007; 8: S3-S21.

3. Ahonen K, Hämäläinen ML, Eerola M, Hoppu K. A randomized trial of rizatriptan in migraine attacks in children. *Neurology* 2006; 67: 1135-1140.

4. Lewis DW, Winner P, Hershey AD, Wasiewski WW. Efficacy of zolmitriptan nasal spray in adolescent migraine. *Pediatrics* 2007; 120: 390-396.

5. Winner P, Rothner AD, Wooten JD, Webster C, Ames M. Sumatriptan nasal spray in adolescent migraineurs: a randomized, double-blind, placebo-controlled, acute study. *Headache* 2006; 46: 212-22.

6. Evers S, Rahmann A, Kraemer C, *et al*. Treatment of childhood migraine attacks with oral zolmitriptan and ibuprofen. *Neurology* 2006; 67: 497-499.

7. Battistella PA, Ruffilli R, Cernetti R, *et al*. A placebo-controlled crossover trial using trazadone in pediatric migraine. *Headache* 1993; 33: 36-39.

8. Hershey AD, Powers SW, Bentti A, Degrauw T. Effectiveness of amitriptyline in the prophylactic management of childhood headache. *Headache* 2000; 40: 539-549.

9. Serdaroglu G, Erhan E, Tekgul H, *et al*. Sodium valproate prophylaxis in childhood migraine. *Headache* 2002; 42: 819-822.

10. Hershey AD, Powers SW, Vockell AB, *et al*. Effectiveness of topiramate in the prevention of childhood headaches. *Headache* 2002; 42: 810-818.

11. Bridge JA, Iyengar S, Salary CB, *et al*. Clinical response and risk for reported suicidal ideation and suicide attempts in pediatric antidepressant treatment: a meta-analysis of randomized controlled trials. *JAMA* 2007; 297: 1683-1696.

12. Sartory G, Muller B, Metsch J, Pothmann R. A comparison of psychological and pharmacological treatment of pediatric migraine. *Behav Res Ther* 1998; 36: 1155-1170.

13. Scharff L, Marcus D, Masek BJ. A controlled study of minimal-contact thermal biofeedback in children with migraine. *J Pediatr Psychol* 2002; 27: 109-119.

14. Isik U, Ersu RH, Ay P, *et al*. Prevalence of headache and its association with sleep disorders in children. *Pediatr Neurol* 2007; 36: 146-151.

15. Gilman DK, Palmero TM, Kabbouche MA, Hershey AD, Powers SW. Primary headache and sleep disturbances in adolescents. *Headache* 2007; 47: 1189-1194.

16. Wang F, Van Den Eeden SK, Ackerson LM, *et al*. Oral magnesium oxide prophylaxis of frequent migrainous headache in children: a randomized, double-blind, placebo-controlled trial. *Headache* 2003; 43: 601-610.

17. Grazzi L, Andrasik F, Usai S, Bussone G. Magnesium as a treatment for paediatric tension-type headache: a clinical replication series. *Neurol Sci* 2005; 25: 338-341.

18. Pothmann R, Danesch U. Migraine prevention in children and adolescents: results of an open study with a special butterbur root extract. *Headache* 2005; 45: 196-203.

19. Marcus DA. Reducing headache disability in children and adolescents. *American Family Physician* 2002; 65: 554-557.

20. Marcus DA. Focus on primary care: diagnosis and management of headache in women. *Obstetrical & Gynecological Survey* 1999; 54: 395-402.
21. Phillips BM. Oral contraceptive drugs and migraine. *Br Med J* 1968; 2: 99.
22. Whitty CM, Hockaday JM. Migraine: a follow-up study of 92 patients. *Br Med J* 1968; 1: 735-736.
23. Kudrow L. The relationship of headache frequency to hormone use in migraine. *Headache* 1975; 15: 36-40.
24. Becker WJ. Use of oral contraceptives in patients with migraine. *Neurology* 1999; 53 (4suppl1): S19-S25.
25. Marcus DA. Headache in pregnancy. *Curr Pain Headache Rep* 2003; 7: 288-296.
26. Francois P, Fabre M, Lioret E, Jan M. Vascular cerebral thrombosis during pregnancy and post-partum. *Neurochirurgie* 2000; 46: 105-109.
27. Lanska DJ, Kryscio RJ. Stroke and intracranial venous thrombosis during pregnancy and puerperium. *Neurology* 1998; 51: 1622-1628.
28. Panagariya A, Maru A. Cerebral venous thrombosis in pregnancy and puerperium - a prospective study. *J Assoc Physicians India* 1997; 45: 857-859.
29. Azpilcueta A, Peral C, Giraldo I, Chen FJ, Contreras G. Meningioma in pregnancy. Report of a case and review of the literature. *Ginecol Obstet Mex* 1995; 63: 349-51.
30. Saitoh Y, Oku Y, Izumoto S, Go J. Rapid growth of a meningioma during pregnancy: relationship with estrogen and progesterone receptors - case report. *Neurol Med Cir* (Tokyo) 1989; 29: 440-3.
31. Arseni C, Simoca I, Jipescu I, Leventi E, Grecu P, Sima A. Pseudotumor cerebri: risk factors, clinical course, prognostic criteria. *Rom J Neurol Psychiatry* 1992; 30: 115-132.
32. Katz VL, Peterson R, Cefalo RC. Pseudotumor cerebri and pregnancy. *Am J Perinatol* 1989; 6: 442-445.
33. Koontz WL, Herbert WP, Cefalo RC. Pseudotumor cerebri in pregnancy. *Obstet Gynecol* 1983; 62: 324-327.
34. Sandrini G, Friberg L, Jänig W, *et al.* Neurophysiological tests and neuroimaging procedures in non-acute headache: guidelines and recommendations. *Eur J Neurol* 2004; 11: 217-224.
35. Levine D, Barnes PD, Edleman RR. Obstetric MR imaging. *Radiology* 1999; 211: 609-17.
36. Baker P, Johnson I, Harvey P, Mansfield P. A three-year follow-up of children imaged *in utero* using echo-planar magnetic resonance. *Am J Obstet Gynecol* 1994; 170: 32-3.
37. Kanal E, Gillen J, Evans J, Savitz D, Shellock F. Survey of reproductive health among female MR workers. *Radiology* 1993; 187: 395-399.
38. ACR standards: MRI safety and sedation. Available at http://acr.org. Accessed March 2008.
39. Dineen R, Banks A, Lenthall R. Imaging of acute neurological conditions in pregnancy and the puerperium. *Clin Radiol* 2005; 60: 1156-1170.
40. Webb JW, Thomsen HS, Morcos SK. The use of iodinated and gadolinium contrast media during pregnancy and lactation. *Eur Radiol* 2005; 15: 1234-1240.

41. Uhl K, Kennedy DL, Kweder SL. Risk management strategies in the Physicians' Desk Reference product labels for pregnancy category X drugs. *Drug Saf* 2002; 25: 885-892.

42. Lo WY, Firedman JM. Teratogenicity of recently introduced medications in human pregnancy. *Obstet Gynecol* 2002; 100: 465-473.

43. Addis A, Sharabi S, Bonati M. Risk classification systems for drug use during pregnancy. Are they a reliable source of information? *Drug Saf* 2000; 23: 245-253.

44. Christian P, West KP, Katz J, *et al.* Cigarette smoking during pregnancy in rural Nepal. Risk factors and effects of beta-carotene and vitamin A supplementation. *Eur J Clin Nutr* 2004; 58: 204-211.

45. Marcus DA, Scharff L, Turk DC. Non-pharmacologial management of headaches during pregnancy. *Psychosom Med* 1995; 57: 527-535.

46. Scharff L, Marcus DA, Turk DC. Maintenance of effects in the non-medical treatment of headaches during pregnancy. *Headache* 1996; 36: 285-290.

47. Gomes KR, Moron AF, Silva R, Siqueira AA. Prevalence of use of medicines during pregnancy and its relationship to maternal factors. *Rev Saude Publica* 1999; 33: 246-254.

48. Damase-Michel C, Lapeyre-Mestre M, Moly C, Fournie A, Montastruc JL. Drug use during pregnancy: survey in 250 women consulting at a university hospital center. *J Gynecol Obstet Biol Repro* (Paris) 2000; 29: 77-85.

49. Fonseca MR, Fonseca E, Bergsten-Mendes G. Prevalence of drug use during pregnancy: a pharmacoepidemiological approach. *Rev Saude Publica* 2002; 36: 205-212.

50. Li DK, Liu L, Odouli R. Exposure to non-steroidal anti-inflammatory drugs during pregnancy and risk of miscarriage: population-based cohort study. *Br Med J* 2003; 327: 368.

51. Kallen B, Lygner PE. Delivery outcome in women who used drugs for migraine during pregnancy with special reference to sumatriptan. *Headache* 2001; 41: 351-356.

52. American College of Obstetricians and Gynecologists. ACOG practice bulletin #52: nausea and vomiting of pregnancy. *Obstet Gynecol* 2004; 103: 803-815.

53. Bayliss H, Churchill D, Beevers M, Beevers DG. Anti-hypertensive drugs in pregnancy and fetal growth: evidence for 'pharmacological programming' in the first trimester? *Hypertens Pregnancy* 2002; 21: 161-174.

54. Sørensen HT, Czeizel AE, Rockerbauer M, Steffensen FH, Olsen J. The risk of limb deficiencies and other congenital malformations in children exposed *in utero* to calcium channel blockers. *Acta Obstet Gynecol Scand* 2001; 80: 397-401.

55. Hemels ME, Einarson A, Koren G, Lanctot KL, Einarson TR. Antidepressant use during pregnancy and the rates of spontaneous abortions: a meta-analysis. *Ann Pharmacother* 2005; 39: 803-809.

56. Bérard A, Ramos E, Rey E, *et al.* First trimester exposure to paroxetine and risk of cardiac malformations in infants: the importance of dosage. *Birth Defects Res B Dev Reprod Toxicol* 2007; 80: 18-27.

57. No authors. Bupropion (amfebutaone): caution during pregnancy. *Prescrire Int* 2005; 14: 225.

58. Chun-Fai-Chan B, Koren G, Fayez I, *et al*. Pregnancy outcome of women exposed to bupropion during pregnancy: a prospective comparative study. *Am J Obstet Gynecol* 2005; 192: 932-936.

59. Montouris G. Gabapentin exposure in human pregnancy: results from the Gabapentin Pregnancy Registry. *Epilepsy Behav* 2003; 4: 310-317.

60. Topiramate (TOPAMAX) prescribing information. In: *Physicians' Desk Reference 2007*. Montvale, NJ: Thomson Healthcare; 2007: 2408.

61. Vila Cerén C, Demestre Guasch X, Raspall Torrent F, *et al*. Topiramate and pregnancy. Neonate with bone anomalies. *An Pediatr (Barc)* 2005; 63: 363-365.

62. American Academy of Pediatric Committee on Drugs. The transfer of drugs and other chemicals into human milk. *Pediatrics* 2001; 108: 776-789.

63. World Health Organization recommendations can be found online at http://www.who.int/child-adolescent-health/. Accessed May 2008.

64. Moses-Kolko EL, Bogen D, Perel J, *et al*. Neonatal signs after late *in utero* exposure to serotonin reuptake inhibitors: literature review and implications for clinical applications. *JAMA* 2005; 293: 2372-2383.

65. Neri I, Granella F, Nappi R, Manzoni GC, Facchinetti F, Genazzani AR. Characteristics of headache at menopause: a clinico-epidemiologic study. *Maturitas* 1993; 17: 31-37.

66. Franceschi M, Colombo B, Rossi P, Canal N. Headache in a population-based elderly cohort. An ancillary study to the Italian Longitudinal Study of Aging (ILAS). *Headache* 1997; 37: 79-82.

67. Wang SJ, Liu HC, Fuh JL, *et al*. Prevalence of headaches in a Chinese elderly population in Kinmen: age and gender effect and cross-cultural comparison. *Neurol* 1997; 49: 195-200.

68. MacGregor EA: 'Menstrual' migraine: towards a definition. *Cephalalgia* 1996; 16: 11-21.

69. Facchinetti F, Nappi RE, Granella F, *et al*. Effects of hormone replacement treatment (HRT) in postmenopausal women with migraine. *Cephalalgia* 2001; 21: 452.

Chapter 9
Emergency department treatment of headache

Introduction

Headache is the fourth most common symptom resulting in emergency department (ED) treatment, accounting for 2.6% of ED visits. As described in Chapter 1, most cases of non-traumatic head pain in the ED are caused by primary, recurring headaches.

Secondary headaches occur less commonly than primary headaches among ED patients reporting non-traumatic headache (see Chapter 1); however, all patients will need a complete history and detailed physical examination to rule out secondary causes of headache. A recent study identified three criteria that successfully predicted significant pathology on neuroimaging (Table 1) [1].

Table 1 Patient features suggesting a need for neuroimaging. (Based on Harris 2000.)

- Glasgow Coma Score <14

- Focal neurology

- Headache with nausea or vomiting

ED treatment of headache includes evaluation for possible secondary headache, symptomatic treatment, and arrangements for follow-up for primary recurring headaches (Table 2). Dehydration has been linked to increased headache activity [2], while increasing water intake decreases headache severity and frequency [3]. Due to the frequent association of nausea and vomiting with headaches that result in an ED visit, the majority of ED headache patients will require rehydration with intravenous fluids. Treating the varied symptoms of non-traumatic headache helps to minimize return visits for insufficiently treated or recurrent headache episodes.

Table 2 General principles for ED treatment of headache.

- Rule out secondary causes of headache

- Treat dehydration

- Treat nausea

- Treat residual pain with headache-specific or general analgesic therapy

- Arrange post-ED follow-up

In general, symptomatic relief should occur within one hour of ED treatment, so most ED studies utilize a one-hour endpoint assessment instead of the typical two-hour assessment used in outpatient headache treatment. This chapter will review data evaluating treatments for non-traumatic headache in the ED.

ED treatment

A survey questioning 105 ED physicians and physician assistants about preferred ED treatments for migraine revealed that most practitioners rely on anti-emetics and analgesics (Figure 1) [4]. Nearly two of every three practitioners also reported using diphenhydramine as adjunctive therapy when using domanergic anti-emetics to minimize akathisia. First-line treatment selection was based on the practitioner's perceptions of likely medication efficacy and availability in the ED. A chart review of 490 ED patients treated with parenteral medication for benign headache confirms a reliance on anti-emetics (Table 3) [5]. Most patients received two medications (82%), with 24% receiving at least three parenteral medications, and 7% treated with at least four parenteral drugs. A subanalysis of patients diagnosed with migraine similarly showed infrequent use of migraine-specific agents (dihydroergotamine in 6% and sumatriptan in 3%), with anti-emetics used for 49%, opioids for 44%, and ketorolac for 16%.

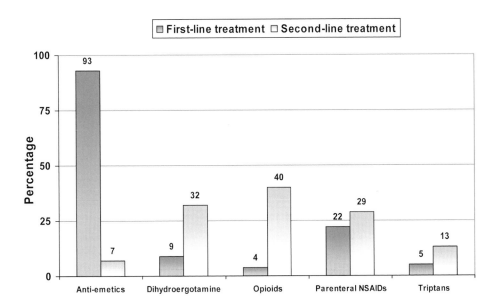

Figure 1 Preferred treatment of migraine by ED practitioners. More than one drug could be identified as first- or second-line therapy. Second-line treatments were used when headache failed to improve with first-line treatment. NSAID=non-steroidal anti-inflammatory drug. (Based on Hurtado 2007.)

Table 3 Most commonly used parenteral medications for benign headache in the ED. (Based on Vinson 2003.)

Drug	Percentage patients receiving
Anti-emetic	
Prochlorperazine	46
Diphenhydramine	37
Promethazine	23
Hydroxyzine	13
Droperidol	8
Metoclopramide	4
Analgesic	
Any opioid	48
Hydromorphone	6
Meperidine	36
Morphine	3
Other opioids	4
Ketorolac	26
Migraine-specific drugs	
Dihydroergotamine	8
Sumatriptan	3
Glucocorticoids	
Dexamethasone	1
Methylprednisolone	0.5

Even though headache is frequently seen in the ED, patients are often under-treated. A prospective survey of adults seen in the ED for non-traumatic headache reported that 34% received no medication or intravenous fluid [6]. Similar to the data reported above, those patients receiving medication were most commonly prescribed anti-emetics or opioids. Two in every three patients had self-medicated prior to the ED visit, usually with a non-opioid analgesic (77%). Only 6% had used a headache-specific treatment, like dihydroergotamine or a triptan. Therefore, pre-ED medications would not have precluded additional treatment in most cases.

Anti-emetic

Both anti-emetics and metoclopramide can effectively relieve severe primary headaches. In a double-blind study, adults presenting to an ED with acute migraine were randomized to receive 10mg prochlorperazine or 20mg metoclopramide [7]. Both drugs were administered intravenously with 25mg intravenous diphenhydramine. Pain relief was achieved by about half of treated patients, with nausea relief in nearly every patient (Figure 2).

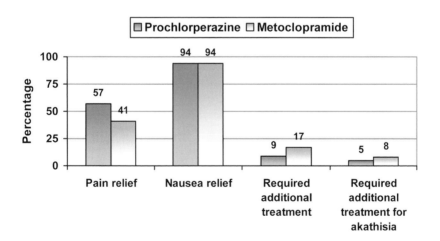

Figure 2 ED treatment with intravenous prochlorperazine vs. metoclopramide. Endpoints were measured two hours after initial treatment. Nausea relief was measured in the 91% of patients who were nauseated at baseline. None of the numeric differences were significant. (Based on Friedman, Esses, in press.)

Although droperidol is less commonly used in ED headache than other anti-emetics, studies report that intramuscular droperidol is more effective in relieving headache-related pain than prochlorperazine [8] and as effective as meperidine [9].

Reported preferences for treating non-traumatic headache with anti-emetics as first-line therapy is supported by retrospective data showing better efficacy in patients treated with metoclopramide compared with hydromorphone (Figure 3) [10]. In all cases, metoclopramide was administered intravenously. Hydromorphone was administered intravenously for 94% and intramuscularly for 6% of patients. Another study similarly reported superior efficacy with metoclopramide compared with pethidine (meperidine) [11].

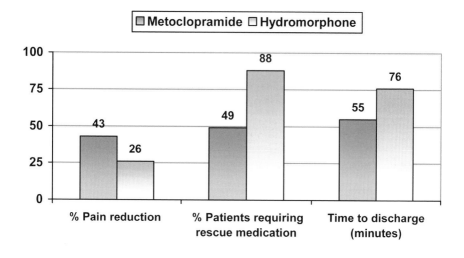

Figure 3 ED treatment with anti-emetic vs. opioid. All differences were significant (P<0.01). (Based on Griffith 2008.)

Anti-emetics have also been directly compared with headache-specific treatment with triptans. In one study, high dose metoclopramide (20mg intravenously, redosed up to four times) was as effective as 6mg subcutaneous sumatriptan [12]. Similarly, the combination of trimethobenzamide plus diphenhydramine was compared with sumatriptan for ED treatment of acute migraine [13]. While short-term relief was superior with sumatriptan, antinausea therapy offered similar 24-hour relief and the authors suggested that antinausea therapy may provide an appropriate acute ED therapy for patients unable to use sumatriptan.

Dihydroergotamine

Dihydroergotamine (DHE) is well established as a successful acute therapy for severe migraine episodes. DHE effectively treats severe, recalcitrant episodes and its long time of action helps to limit recurrence among patients with typically long-lasting attacks.

DHE was tested against opioids in a double-blind study in which adults with acute migraine in the ED were randomized to receive intramuscular injections of 1mg DHE or 1.5mg/kg meperidine (Figure 4) [14]. Both groups received concomitant therapy with hydroxyzine. Patients receiving either treatment experienced similar improvement in migraine symptoms, although recurrence was more common in patients receiving meperidine.

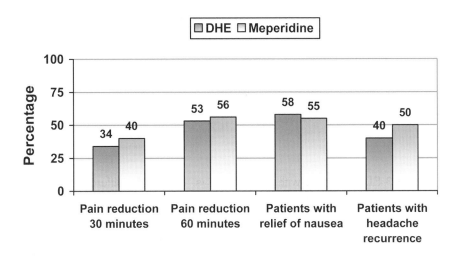

Figure 4 Intramuscular DHE vs. meperidine for ED migraine in adults (Based on Carleton 1998.)

Magnesium

Intravenous magnesium sulphate may also be used in the ED treatment of migraine, with efficacy shown using 1g intravenously [15]. In a randomized, prospective study, 2g intravenous magnesium sulphate was as effective as 10mg intravenous metoclopramide and more effective than placebo [16].

Non-opioid analgesics

Intravenous ketorolac may provide a non-opioid ED option for severe headache; however, controlled studies consistently show inferior efficacy

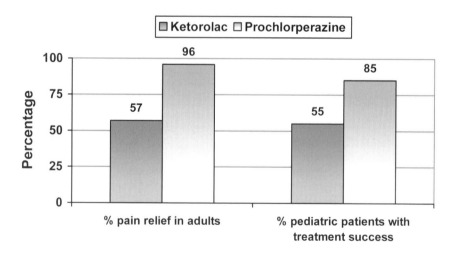

Figure 5 ED treatment with ketorolac vs prochlorperazine. All patients were randomly assigned to double-blind intravenous treatment with ketorolac (30mg in adults and 0.5mg/kg to a maximum dose of 30mg in children) or prochlorperazine (10mg in adults or 0.15mg/kg to a maximum dose of 10mg in children). Successful treatment in children was defined as a headache reduction of at least 50%. Numerical differences were significant at P<0.05. (Based on Seim 1998 and Brousseau 2004.)

compared with anti-emetics in both adults and children (Figure 5) [17, 18]. Intravenous ketorolac did produce a superior reduction in migraine pain in adults randomized to 30mg ketorolac versus 20mg intranasal sumatriptan (77% vs. 27%, P<0.05) [19].

A slow infusion of 100mg tramadol in 100mL saline versus placebo in a single-blind, randomized study resulted in significantly better pain relief after one hour than placebo (71% vs. 35%, P<0.05) [20]. Headache recurrence was similar for both groups. Figure 6 shows pain reduction in adults seeking ED treatment for migraine after being randomized to double-blind, intramuscular treatment with 100mg tramadol or 75mg diclofenac [21]. A response occurred earlier with diclofenac. A two-hour reduction in headache, photophobia, phonophobia, and nausea were similar with either treatment. Rescue treatment at two hours was used by 20% of patients receiving either treatment.

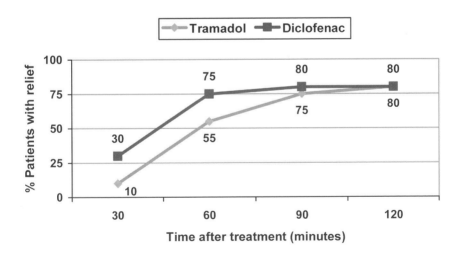

Figure 6 ED migraine treatment with intramuscular tramadol vs. non-steroidal anti-inflammatory drug. (Based on Engindeniz 2005.)

Opioid analgesics

While opioid analgesics are widely used for headache treatment in the ED, their efficacy as headache-relieving treatment is inferior to other medications, such as anti-emetics. Consequently, opioids are most appropriately used as rescue rather than first-line headache treatment. Furthermore, caution should be exercised when administering potential medications of abuse such as opioids. Self-report of ongoing problems with substances of abuse are often unreliable. In one survey, 17% of patients seeking opioid treatment in the ED for headache tested positive on urine screens for drugs of abuse that they failed to report they had taken [22]. Identified substances were benzodiazepines, marijuana, and cocaine.

Steroid

Dexamethasone has minimal efficacy in most patients receiving ED treatment of migraine, although benefit has been shown in patients with migraine lasting >72 hours [23]. Double-blind, placebo-controlled studies have evaluated the benefit of adjunctive steroid treatment to reduce headache recurrence after treatment in the ED. Treatment with either oral or intravenous dexamethasone fails to reduce migraine recurrence [24-27].

Sumatriptan

Despite limited use in the ED, subcutaneous sumatriptan provides an effective and well tolerated treatment for primary headache. A prospective study evaluated the outcome of 147 patients with a primary headache (88% migraine and 12% tension-type headache) treated with 6mg sumatriptan subcutaneously [28]. Half of all patients experienced a significant reduction in symptoms after 30 minutes, with a response in nearly 60% after one hour (Figure 7). One in three patients required additional therapy after one hour, most commonly an anti-emetic or opioid. Response was similar for patients with either a migraine or tension-type headache.

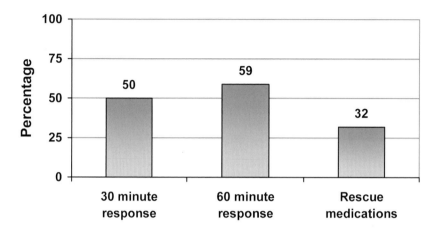

Figure 7 ED response to primary headache treatment with sumatriptan. Graph shows percentage of patients experiencing a reduction in headache severity of at least 50% and the percentage of patients using rescue medications at 60 minutes. (Based on Miner 2007.)

Valproate

Intravenous valproate offers an effective alternative acute migraine treatment in patients who are not pregnant and are using adequate contraception. A small study treating 40 migraine patients intravenously with 500mg valproate versus 10mg prochlorperazine, each diluted in 10mL saline and administered over two minutes, showed better success with prochlorperazine, with additional rescue therapy required in 79% treated with valproate versus 25% with prochlorperazine [29].

In an open-label study, acute migraine patients were randomized to receive intravenous valproate or intramuscular dihydroergotamine with metoclopramide [30]. One hour after treatment, pain and nausea decreased with both treatments although photophobia and phonophobia persisted (Figure 8). While early treatment response was similar, sustained relief was better with dihydroergotamine with metoclopramide. Twenty-four hours after treatment, a moderate to severe headache was reported by 40% with valproate and 10% with dihydroergotamine with metoclopramide. None of the valproate-treated patients reported medication side effects, while 15% of the dihydroergotamine with metoclopramide group reported nausea and diarrhea during the first four hours after treatment.

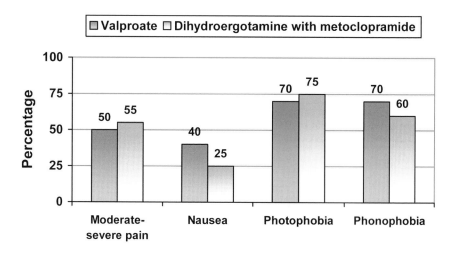

Figure 8 Migraine symptoms reported one hour post-treatment with valproate or dihydroergotamine plus metoclopramide. All differences were significant (P<0.01). (Based on Edwards 2001.)

Post-ED treatment

Following ED treatment for headache, post-ED treatment recommendations should be provided, including for patients who achieved successful headache relief (Table 4). Despite the recurrent nature of most non-traumatic headaches seen in the ED, patients often receive only limited recommendations for the treatment of recurring or future headaches or follow-up care plans. A survey of adults receiving ED treatment for a chief complaint of non-traumatic headache reported that, although only 22% were pain-free at the time of leaving the ED, discharge medications were provided to only 37% of patients (Figure 9) [6]. Only 41% of patients were advised to arrange follow-up with a physician for headache management and headache recurred within 24 hours of ED treatment for two of every three patients. Failure to provide comprehensive post-ED treatment recommendations can result in unnecessary headache disability and future ED visits for treatment of benign headache.

Table 4 Post-ED treatment recommendations.

- Anti-emetic

- Non-steroidal anti-inflammatory drug

- Triptan

- Opioid analgesic

- Referral to PCP or headache specialist

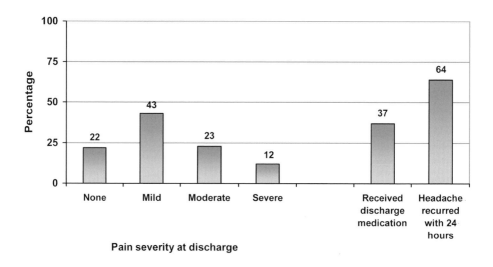

Figure 9 Post-ED headache treatment. (Based on Gupta 2007.)

Conclusions

All patients seeking ED treatment for headache should be evaluated for possible secondary headache. First-line treatment for patients with a non-traumatic, primary headache includes rehydration and anti-emetics. Patients with residual headache symptoms may need additional treatment with headache-specific therapies (i.e., triptans or dihydroergotamine) or non-opioid analgesics. Additional options include intravenous magnesium, intravenous valproate, and opioids. Steroids offer minimal benefit.

Key Summary

◆ ED headache treatment focuses on ruling out secondary causes of headaches, treating dehydration, pain, and nausea, and providing post-ED care.

◆ Anti-emetics are the preferred first-line ED headache treatment.

◆ Anti-emetics can effectively relieve both headache-related pain and nausea.

◆ Headache-related pain can be effectively relieved with headache-specific treatments or non-specific analgesics.

◆ Headache recurs within 24 hours of ED treatment for two in every three patients, necessitating the provision of post-ED headache care instructions. The likelihood of recurrence is similar after most headache treatments, with a lower recurrence rate with dihydroergotamine.

References

1. Harris JE, Draper HL, Rhodes AI, Stevens JM. High yield criteria for emergency cranial computed tomography in adult patients with no history of head injury. *J Accid Emerg Med* 2000; 17: 15-17.

2. Blau JN. Water deprivation: a new migraine precipitant. *Headache* 2005; 45: 757-759.

3. Spigt MG, Kuijper EC, Schayck CP, *et al.* Increasing daily water intake for prophylactic treatment of headache: a pilot trial. *Eur J Neurol* 2005; 12: 715-718.

4. Hurtado TR, Vinson DR, Vandenberg JT. ED treatment of migraine headache: factors influencing pharmacotherapeutic choices. *Headache* 2007; 47: 1134-1143.

5. Vinson DR, Hurtado TR, Vandenberg JT, Banwart L. Variations among emergency departments in the treatment of benign headache. *Ann Emerg Med* 2003; 41: 90-97.

6. Gupta MX, Silberstein SD, Young WB, *et al.* Less is not more: underutilization of headache medications in a university hospital emergency department. *Headache* 2007; 47: 1125-1133.

7. Friedman BW, Esses D, Solorzano C, et al. A randomized controlled trial of prochlorperazine versus metoclopramide for treatment of acute migraine. *Ann Emerg Med*, in press.

8. Miner JR, Fish SJ, Smith SW, Biros MH. Droperidol vs. prochlorperazine for benign headaches in the emergency department. *Acad Emerg Med* 2001; 8: 873-879.

9. Richman PB, Allegra J, Eskin B, et al. A randomized clinical trial to assess the efficacy of intramuscular droperidol for the treatment of acute migraine. *Am J Emerg Med* 2002; 20: 39-42.

10. Griffith JD, Mycyk MB, Kyriacou DN. Metoclopramide versus hydromorphone for the emergency department treatment of migraine headache. *J Pain* 2008; 9: 88-94.

11. Cicek M, Karcioglu O, Pariak I, et al. Prospective, randomized, double-blind, controlled comparison of metoclopramide and pethidine in the emergency treatment of acute primary vascular and tension-type headache episodes. *Emerg Med J* 2004; 21: 323-326.

12. Friedman BW, Corbo J, Lipton RB. A trial of metoclopramide vs sumatriptan for the emergency department treatment of migraines. *Neurology* 2005; 64: 463-468.

13. Friedman BW, Hockberg M, Esses D, et al. A clinical trial of trimethobenzamide/diphenhydramine versus sumatriptan for acute migraine. *Headache* 2006; 46: 934-941.

14. Carleton SG, Shesser RF, Pietrzak MP, et al. Double-blind, multicenter trial to compare the efficacy of intramuscular dihydroergotmaine plus hydroxyzine versus intramuscular meperidine plus hydroxyzine for the emergency department treatment of acute migraine headache. *Ann Emerg Med* 1998; 32: 129-138.

15. Bigal ME, Bordini CA, Tepper SJ, Speciali JG. Intravenous magnesium sulphate in the acute treatment of migraine without aura and migraine with aura. A randomized, double-blind, placebo-controlled study. *Cephalalgia* 2002; 22: 345-353.

16. Cete Y, Dora B, Ertan C, Ozdemir C, Oktay C. A randomized prospective placebo-controlled study of intravenous magnesium sulphate vs. metoclopramide in the management of acute migraine attacks in the Emergency Department. *Cephalalgia* 2005; 25: 199-204.

17. Seim MB, March JA, Dunn KA. Intravenous ketorolac vs intravenous prochlorperazine for the treatment of migraine headaches. *Acad Emerg Med* 1998; 5: 573-576.

18. Brousseau DC, Duffy SJ, Anderson AC, Linakis JG. Treatment of pediatric migraine headaches: a randomized, double-blind trial of prochlorperazine versus ketorolac. *Ann Emerg Med* 2004; 43: 256-262.

19. Meredith JT, Wait S, Brewer KL. A prospective double-blind study of nasal sumatriptan versus IV ketorolac in migraine. *Am J Emerg Med* 2003; 21: 173-175.

20. Alemdar M, Pekdemir M, Selekler HM. Single-dose intravenous tramadol for acute migraine pain in adults: a single-blind, prospective, randomized, placebo-controlled clinical trial. *Clin Ther* 2007; 29: 1441-1447.

21. Engindeniz Z, Demircan C, Karli N, et al. Intramuscular tramadol vs. diclofenac sodium for the treatment of acute migraine attacks in emergency department: a prospective, randomized, double-blind study. *J Headache Pain* 2005; 6: 143-148.

22. Schuckman H, Hazelett S, Powell C, Steer S. A validation of self-reported substance use with biochemical testing among patients presenting to the emergency department seeking treatment for backache, headache, and toothache. *Subst Use Misuse* 2008; 43: 589-595.
23. Friedman BW, Greenwald P, Bania TC, *et al*. Randomized trial of IV dexamethasone for acute migraine in the emergency department. *Neurology* 2007; 69: 2038-2044.
24. Kelly AM, Kerr D, Clooney M. Impact of oral dexamethasone versus placebo after ED treatment of migraine with phenothiazines on the rate of recurrent headache: a randomized controlled trial. *Emerg Med J* 2008; 25: 26-29.
25. Friedman BW, Greenwald P, Bania, *et al*. Randomized trial of IV dexamethasone for acute migraine in the emergency department. *Neurology* 2007; 69: 2038-2044.
26. Rowe BH, Colman I, Edmonds ML, *et al*. Randomized controlled trial of intravenous dexamethasone to prevent relapse in acute migraine headache. *Headache* 2008; 28: 333-340.
27. Donaldson D, Sundermann R, Jackson R, Bastani A. Intravenous dexamethasone vs placebo as adjunctive therapy to reduce the recurrence rate of acute migraine headaches: a multicenter, double-blind, placebo-controlled randomized clinical trial. *Am J Emerg Med* 2008; 26: 124-30.
28. Miner JR, Smith SW, Moore J, Biros M. Sumatriptan for the treatment of undifferentiated primary headaches in the ED. *Am J Emerg Med* 2007; 25: 60-64.
29. Tanen DA, Miller S, French T, Riffenburgh RH. Intravenous sodium valproate versus prochlorperazine for the emergency department treatment of acute migraine headaches: a prospective, randomized, double-blind trial. *Ann Emerg Med* 2003; 41: 847-853.
30. Edwards KR, Norton J, Behnke M. Comparison of intravenous valproate versus intramuscular dihydroergotamine and metoclopramide for acute treatment of migraine headaches. *Headache* 2001; 41: 976-980.

Chapter 10
Uncommon and geriatric headaches

Introduction

As described earlier, most patients seeking treatment for headaches will be diagnosed with commonly occurring primary headaches, such as migraine, tension-type headaches, and cluster headaches, or typical secondary headaches, like post-traumatic headache or headache related to viral illness or another readily identified condition. In rare cases, patients describe unusual headache patterns. This chapter will describe features of uncommon headaches and headaches unique to older adults.

Uncommon headaches

Uncommon headaches affect <1% of the population, with limited epidemiological data available for a number of these conditions. In many cases, information is restricted to series of case reports rather than assessments of large population samples to determine incidence, prevalence, and important demographic factors. Although each uncommon headache disorder is characterized by distinctive features, these conditions occur infrequently and patients for whom these diagnoses are considered should first undergo a thorough assessment, including neuroimaging, prior to assigning any of these diagnoses. Remember - patients are more likely to present with an unusual or atypical presentation of a common disorder than a characteristic presentation of a rare headache condition.

Basilar migraine

Basilar migraine is a type of migraine in which aura symptoms can be referred to neurological functions supplied by the brainstem or bilateral cerebral hemispheres (Table 1). More than one symptom is needed for an aura to result in the classification of basilar migraine, particularly as anxiety and hyperventilation often result in the occurrence of a single one of these symptoms, especially hand paresthesia or dizziness. Motor deficits are characteristically absent in basilar migraine and, if present, often represent hemiplegic migraine. Epidemiological data are sparse, due to controversies in diagnostic criteria; however, basilar migraine is mostly seen in adolescent girls.

Table 1 Aura symptoms of basilar migraine. Patients need to have at least two of these features during a single aura.

- Ataxia

- Bilateral sensory disturbance

- Blindness, double vision, or bilateral visual symptoms

- Dysarthria

- Hearing loss

- Loss of consciousness

- Tinnitus

- Vertigo

Due to the disabling nature of the aura symptoms of basilar migraine, patients with this type of headache are generally treated with prevention therapies. Patients with basilar migraine have been excluded from clinical trials testing headache-specific therapies, like the triptans; consequently, triptans are currently considered to be contraindicated for basilar migraine patients. Reports of good efficacy and tolerability with triptans in small numbers of patients with basilar migraine suggest that restrictions in this population may have been overstated [1].

Benign intracranial hypertension

Benign intracranial hypertension was previously referred to as pseudotumor cerebri and describes markedly increased intracranial pressure unrelated to inflammatory or structural pathology. The overall population incidence of benign intracranial hypertension is about five cases per 100,000 persons [2]. Surveys of patients with benign intracranial hypertension in both Europe and the United States show remarkably similar patient demographics, with most patients being obese women of reproductive age (Table 2) [2, 3]. Characteristics are described in Table 3. Opening cerebrospinal fluid pressure is used to confirm intracranial hypertension, with indicative pressures varying by age (Table 4) [4].

Table 2 Typical patient with benign intracranial hypertension. (Based on Galvin 2004 and Asensio-Sánchez 2007.)

- Female gender - 90-92%

- Mean age - 34 years

- Obesity - 88-100%

Table 3 Characteristics of benign intracranial hypertension.

- Diffuse, constant headache

- Aggravated by maneuvers that increase intracranial pressure
  - Coughing
  - Straining or Valsalva
  - Rising from sitting with the development of transient visual obscurations

- Increased intracranial pressure, as evidenced by
  - Papilledema
  - Enlarged blind spot
  - Sixth nerve palsy
  - Markedly increased pressure reading on lumbar puncture (Table 4)   with normal spinal fluid chemistry and cell count

- Symptomatic relief after reduction in intracranial pressure through spinal fluid drainage

Table 4 Typical spinal fluid opening pressure in patients with benign intracranial hypertension.

- Children <8 years old: >180 mm H_2O

- Children ≥8 years old: >250 mm H_2O

- Adults: >250 mm H_2O

In many cases, benign intracranial hypertension has been linked to endocrine or hormonal dysfunction or medication exposure (Table 5). Patients presenting with benign intracranial hypertension should be evaluated for the presence of and treated for these conditions.

Table 5 Conditions associated with benign intracranial hypertension.

- Addison's disease

- Dural sinus thrombosis

- Hyperparathyroidism

- Hypervitaminosis A

- Menarche

- Obesity or recent weight gain

- Phenothiazine treatment

- Polycystic ovarian syndrome

- Pregnancy

- Steroid treatment or withdrawal

- Tetracycline treatment

Treatment includes correction of any underlying predisposing conditions. In most cases, weight loss will be recommended. Acetazolamide to reduce spinal fluid production and draining of spinal fluid with repeated lumbar punctures often decrease symptoms. All patients will require regular monitoring by a neurologist and ophthalmologist. Lumboperitoneal or ventriculoperitoneal shunting or optic nerve sheath fenestration may become necessary to protect patients from permanent visual loss.

Hemicrania continua

As described by the name, patients with hemicrania continua experience a persistent, continuous, unilateral headache (Table 6). Hemicrania continua responds to treatment with indomethacin, which confirms the diagnosis.

Table 6 Features of hemicrania continua.

---

* Unilateral pain always affecting the same side of the head

* Pain is continuous

* Accompanied by unilateral autonomic features
  - Lacrimation
  - Miosis
  - Ptosis
  - Rhinorrhea

* Responsive to indomethacin

Response to indomethacin provides diagnostic confirmation and also an ongoing effective treatment. Patients unable to tolerate indomethacin may respond to topiramate [5].

Hemiplegic migraine

Hemiplegic migraine may occur as a familial or sporadic condition and has been estimated to affect about 0.01% of the population [6]. The genetics of familial hemiplegic migraine are described in Chapter 4. Aura symptoms suggesting basilar migraine occur in nearly two of every three patients with familial hemiplegic migraine. Patients with hemiplegic migraine experience an aura that includes transient motor weakness plus visual phenomena (e.g., areas of visual loss or visual hallucinations like flickering lights, spots or lines), sensory symptoms (e.g., numbness or paresthesias), or dysphasia. Familial hemiplegic migraine type 1 has been linked to mutations on chromosome 19 and migraine episode features may include confusion and loss of consciousness.

The treatment of hemiplegic migraine is generally the same as for other types of migraine headache. Similar to basilar migraine, patients with hemiplegic migraine have been excluded from clinical trials testing triptans, which are, therefore, considered to be contraindicated in patients with hemiplegic migraine. Reports of good efficacy and tolerability with triptans in small numbers of patients with hemiplegic migraine suggest that contraindications in this population may have been overstated [7, 8].

Paroxysmal hemicrania

This headache shares features with cluster headaches, with brief, severe, unilateral pain typically around the eye. Contrary to cluster headaches, however, females are predominantly affected by paroxysmal hemicrania and pain episodes are very short in duration and recur more frequently throughout the day (Table 7). Patients (especially females) with frequent episodes of short-duration cluster-like headaches may be treated with indomethacin to complete the diagnosis. As for cluster headaches, paroxysmal hemicrania may also be experienced as an episodic condition with a cluster of attacks separated by prolonged asymptomatic periods or a chronic condition without prolonged remission periods.

Response to indomethacin provides diagnostic confirmation and also an ongoing effective treatment. Patients unable to tolerate indomethacin may respond to topiramate [9].

Table 7 Features of paroxysmal hemicrania.

- Severe, unilateral orbital, peri-orbital, or temporal pain

- Pain episodes last several to 30 minutes

- Accompanied by unilateral autonomic features
  - Facial/orbital edema
  - Lacrimation
  - Miosis
  - Ptosis
  - Rhinorrhea

- >5 episodes daily

- Responsive to indomethacin

Short-lasting unilateral neuralgiform headache with conjunctival injection and tearing (SUNCT)

As described by its name, patients with SUNCT experience short-duration, unilateral head pain associated with marked, unilateral redness and tearing of the eye on the same side as the pain. Episodes typically last a few seconds to a few minutes and are repeated many times throughout the day.

Patients lacking the combination of conjunctival injection and tearing may be diagnosed with short-lasting unilateral neuralgiform headache attacks with cranial autonomic symptoms (SUNA). SUNA attacks are similarly of a short duration, with repeated attacks of unilateral orbital or peri-orbital pain and may be associated with a variety of autonomic features including:

◆ conjunctival injection;
◆ eyelid edema;
◆ lacrimation;
◆ rhinorrhea.

A survey of patients with SUNCT (N=43) and SUNA (N=9) reported autonomic symptoms more commonly with SUNCT than SUNA (Table 8) [10]. The average length of attacks was one minute, with a range of one second to ten minutes. The number of attacks per day ranged from two to hundreds. Symptoms were triggered by cutaneous stimulation in 79% of SUNCT and 33% of SUNA patients, most commonly by touching the face or chewing.

Table 8 Prevalence of autonomic symptoms (%).

Autonomic symptom	SUNCT	SUNA
Conjunctival injection	100	22
Lacrimation	100	44
Nasal blockage	40	22
Rhinorrhea	53	22
Edema	49	11
Ptosis	51	33
Facial flushing	9	11
Sweating	7	11

A second report of the same 52 patients described above reported effective treatment with intravenous lidocaine at 1.5-3.5mg/kg/hour as an acute therapy [11]. Effective prevention treatments included lamotrigine (dosed to a maximum of 400mg daily), topiramate (maximum 400mg daily), and gabapentin (maximum 3600mg daily). Another report of 24 subjects with SUNCT or SUNA reported good efficacy with subcutaneous lignocaine and lamotrigine [12].

Geriatric headaches

Although headaches tend to diminish with age, one in five seniors reports recurring headaches. Three or more headache episodes during the preceding year were reported by 22% of 1031 community-dwelling adults of 65 years or older [13]. Similar to younger population samples, headache prevalence was higher in elderly women. Migraine was particularly sensitive to reduction with advancing age, with a lower prevalence when compared with a similar survey of young adults (Figure 1) [14].

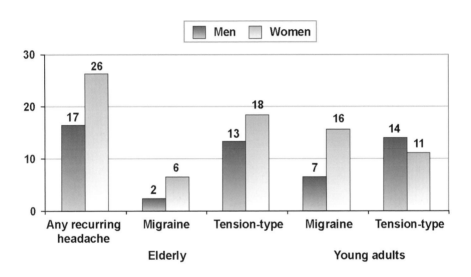

Figure 1 Prevalence of recurring headache in the elderly (mean age = 75 years) and young adults (mean age = 22 years). (Based on Camarda 2003 and Deleu 2001.)

New onset, primary headache is unusual in older adults, with most new headaches caused by another condition. Primary headaches seen in young adults, like migraine, uncommonly begin after age 50. Headache may be related to medication side effects, arthritis in the cervical spine, inflammation or infection, an intracranial mass, or other pathology. In most cases, seniors reporting new onset headache or a change in headache pattern will require radiographic study and often blood work to rule out giant cell arteritis. Several more common headache conditions in elderly patients are described below.

Giant cell arteritis

Definition and epidemiology

Giant cell arteritis (also called temporal arteritis) is an inflammatory condition that typically occurs at or after age 50, with most affected individuals >70 years old [15]. The incidence is about 19 cases per 100,000 persons ≥50 years old, with women affected over twice as often as men [16]. Giant cell arteritis may occur as an isolated head pain syndrome (Table 9) or a symptom of polymyalgia rheumatica (Table 10) [17].

Table 9 Prevalence of symptoms in patients with giant cell arteritis (Based on Salvarani 2002.)

- Head pain/scalp tenderness - 66%

- Fatigue with chewing (jaw claudication) - 50%

- Polymyalgia rheumatica - 40%

- Visual loss/disturbance - 20%

- Low grade fever - 15%

- Cough - 10%

Table 10 Prevalence of symptoms in patients with polymyalgia rheumatica (Based on Salvarani 2002.)

- Giant cell arteritis - 16-21%

- Proximal limb pain and stiffness
  - 70-95% shoulders
  - 50-70% hip and neck

- Distal extremity symptoms - 50%
  - Asymmetrical arthritis in the wrists and knees
  - Carpal tunnel syndrome
  - Edema in the hands and feet

- Systemic symptoms - 30%
  - Anorexia
  - Fatigue
  - Fever
  - Weight loss

Giant cell arteritis is a medical emergency that should be considered in the differential diagnosis of any new headache in elderly patients because of the significant risk for vision loss and stroke. Visual symptoms occur in 30% of patients with biopsy-proven giant cell arteritis, with permanent partial or total visual loss occurring in 19%, most commonly due to anterior ischemic neuropathy (92%) and, less commonly, central retinal artery occlusion (8%) [18]. Visual loss is unilateral for three of every four patients. Stroke, usually in the vertebrobasilar distribution, occurs in approximately 3% of giant cell arteritis patients [19].

Assessment and treatment

Evaluation begins with blood work to determine the hematocrit and erythrocyte sedimentation rate (ESR) or C-reactive protein. Patients with a strong presumptive diagnosis of giant cell arteritis or anterior ischemic neuropathy should be treated with steroids presumptively, immediately after blood work has been obtained. Treatment should not be delayed until blood test results or a temporal artery biopsy has been obtained. Biopsy should, however, be performed within two to three days of initiating steroid therapy.

Glucocorticoids are first-line treatment for giant cell arteritis, effectively relieving clinical symptoms and preventing ischemic complications in most patients (Table 11) [20]. The tapering schedule is dependent on continuation of symptomatic control and reduction in the ESR. Small increases in the ESR often occur during steroid tapering and do not require an increase in steroids if the patient remains asymptomatic. Because treatment is started before a diagnosis is verified, long-term steroid treatment should not be utilized in patients in whom the diagnosis has been ruled out (e.g., negative ESR and negative biopsy). Glucocorticoid complications occur frequently (Table 12) [21]. Non-steroid treatment has been tested with methotrexate, azathioprine, anti-tumor necrosis factor-α monoclonal antibody infliximab, and low-dose aspirin; however, controlled trial data are sparse and inconsistent [20].

Table 11 Treatment regimen for giant cell arteritis.

- Initiate treatment with oral steroids (e.g., prednisone 60-100mg daily) if no visual symptoms

- Initiate treatment with intravenous steroids (e.g., 1000mg methylprenisolone daily pulsed in 2-4 divided doses for several days) if visual symptoms are present

- Anticipate headache resolution within several days of initiating steroids

- Continue oral steroids, tapering over the first month (e.g., 40mg prednisone daily after 4 weeks)

- Continue lower dose oral steroid for 6-18 months, decreasing dosage by 10% per week or 2.5 to 5.0mg every 1 to 2 weeks until a maintenance dosage of 10-20mg/day is reached

Table 12 Incidence of steroid-related complications with treatment for giant cell arteritis. (Based on Proven 2003.)

- Any glucocorticoid side effect - 86%

- Posterior subcapsular cataract - 41%

- Any fracture - 38%
  - Vertebral fracture - 23%
  - Hip fracture - 16%

- Infection - 31%

- Hypertension - 22%

- Diabetes - 9%

- Gastrointestinal bleeding - 4%

Hypnic headache

Hypnic headache is a rare primary headache that begins after 50 years of age. Similar to cluster headaches, patients with hypnic headache (also dubbed 'alarm clock headache') awake predictably with short-duration night-time headaches (Table 13). Unlike cluster headaches, the pain of

Table 13 Characteristics of hypnic headache.

- Occurs during sleep

- At least 15 episodes per month

- Pain is bilateral or diffuse

- Pain lasts a few minutes up to 3 hours

- No associated autonomic symptoms

- Secondary headache has been excluded

hypnic headaches is more diffuse and not associated with autonomic features like rhinorrhea or lacrimation. This diagnosis should only be made after evaluation has ruled out secondary causes of headache.

A review of 71 case reports of hypnic headache in the literature resulted in a description of typical features (Table 14) [22]. Associated nausea occurred in one in every five patients. Photophobia, phonophobia, and autonomic features were infrequently endorsed. Treatment results from these cases suggested that the most effective treatments are acetylsalicylic acid for acute therapy and lithium for prevention. Indomethacin was noted to benefit those patients with exclusively unilateral attacks.

Table 14 Typical features of hypnic headaches. (Based on Evers 2003.)

Characteristic	Number
Mean age at onset	63 years
Female:male ratio	2:1
Pain location (%)	
• Unilateral	39
• Bilateral	61
Pain description (%)	
• Dull	57
• Throbbing	38
• Sharp or stabbing	5
Pain severity (%)	
• Mild	2
• Moderate	68
• Severe	31

Post-herpetic neuralgia

Definition and epidemiology

Post-herpetic neuralgia is defined as pain that persists >1 month after the onset of shingles or herpes zoster. Post-herpetic neuralgia most commonly affects the trunk or face (especially the ophthalmic division of the trigeminal nerve) [23]. Risk factors for the development of post-herpetic neuralgia include female gender, older age, experiencing pain or sensory disturbance before the development of the rash, a greater pain severity during acute herpes zoster, and a larger distribution for the zoster rash [24]. Post-herpetic neuralgia occurs in one in three patients following acute zoster and lasts one year in approximately one in ten patients (Figure 2) [25]. Post-herpetic neuralgia is more likely to persist in older patients and those with more severe pain symptoms.

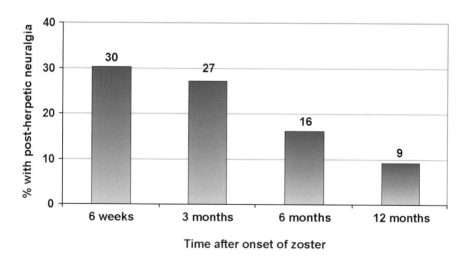

Figure 2 Prevalence of post-herpetic neuralgia in patients developing herpes zoster. (Based on Scott 2003.)

Prevention and treatment

Zoster vaccination of immunocompetent seniors with a history of varicella was shown to reduce the incidence of shingles by 51% and post-herpetic neuralgia by 66% in the large, double-blind Shingles Prevention Trial [26]. Consequently, the Centers for Disease Control and Prevention Advisory Committee on Immunization Practices recommend vaccinating all seniors >60 years old for the prevention of herpes zoster and subsequent post-herpetic neuralgia, unless otherwise contraindicated [27]. Vaccinating all 60-year-olds has been estimated to be able to reduce the number of patients with herpes zoster in the United States by about 250,000 cases annually, as well as a comparably substantial number of patients who would be spared from developing post-herpetic neuralgia [28].

Among patients who develop herpes zoster, the risk for developing post-herpetic neuralgia and subsequent duration of post-herpetic neuralgia may be reduced by early and aggressive treatment with antiviral therapy (Table 15) [29-32]. The incidence of post-herpetic neuralgia may also be decreased by early treatment with neuropathic medication. For example, low-dose amitriptyline (25mg/day) administered within 48 hours of the onset of the zoster rash significantly reduces post-herpetic neuralgia (Figure 3) [33].

Table 15 Antiviral therapy for early herpes zoster (within 72 hours of symptom onset).

• Acyclovir

• Famciclovir

• Valacyclovir

• Brivudin (not available in the United States)

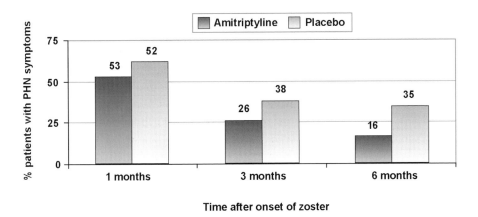

Figure 3 Post-herpetic neuralgia (PHN) after acute zoster treated within 48 hours of rash onset with amitriptyline or placebo. Differences between amitriptyline and placebo are significant (P<0.05). (Based on Bowsher 1997.)

Once patients have developed post-herpetic neuralgia, an evidence-based consensus statement from the American Academy of Neurology recommends treatment with [34]:

◆ tricyclic antidepressants;
◆ gabapentin;
◆ pregabalin;
◆ a lidocaine patch;
◆ opioids.

Inflammation and increased prostaglandin activity occur in early post-herpetic neuralgia, suggesting a possible role for anti-inflammatory therapy [35]. In one study, treatment with topical aspirin (750-1500mg plus 20-30mL diethyl ether), but not other non-steroidal anti-inflammatory drugs, reduced pain more than placebo (66% with aspirin vs 34% with placebo) [36]. Pain relief occurred rapidly (approximately four minutes) and persisted for a mean of 3.6 hours.

Trigeminal neuralgia

Definition and epidemiology

Trigeminal neuralgia is an excruciating, lancinating facial pain, typically triggered by stimulating the skin over the affected area, such as by touching, talking, or chewing (Table 16). Patients sometimes also report a dull facial pain between severe paroxysms. Pain most commonly affects the second or third divisions of the trigeminal nerve. The overall incidence of trigeminal neuralgia in the general population is 0.004% [37]. A recent review of primary care patients reported 27 incident cases per 100,000 person-years [38]. Risk increases with age and women are twice as likely to be affected as men.

Table 16 Typical characteristics of trigeminal neuralgia.

* Lancinating facial pain

* Usually affecting cheek and jaw

* More often affecting right side of face

* Pain triggered by tactile stimulation or facial movement

Treatment

Trigeminal neuralgia is initially treated conservatively (Table 17). While oxcarbazepine is generally less effective than carbamazepine, tolerability is typically superior [39]. Phenytoin is less well tolerated; however, patients can achieve effective blood levels more quickly by using initial loading doses. Baclofen is likewise consistently effective for trigeminal neuralgia. Gabapentin and pregabalin are less effective, but well tolerated. A review of 92 patients with trigeminal neuralgia being treated with gabapentin showed complete or nearly complete pain relief in 27% and partial pain relief in 20%; pain relief was sustained in 63% [40]. Recently, open-label treatment with pregabalin 150-600mg daily showed significant pain relief after eight weeks in 49% of patients, with complete pain relief in 25% [41]. Among patients experiencing early pain relief, relief lasted for one year in 85%. Patients often experience pain-free periods lasting months to years, so medication taper may be attempted after the patient has been pain-free for several months.

Table 17 Medication therapy for trigeminal neuralgia.

- First-line
  - Carbamazepine
  - Oxcarbazepine
  - Phenytoin
  - Baclofen

- Second-line
  - Gabapentin
  - Pregabalin

Patients failing to achieve or maintain adequate pain control with medication therapy may be treated with percutaneous retrogasserian glycerol rhizotomy, stereotactic (gamma knife) radiosurgery, or microvascular decompression (Table 18) [42-46]. Retromastoid microvascular decompression cushions the trigeminal nerve by placing a pad between the trigeminal nerve near its root and nearby blood vessels. Microvascular decompression offers the most complete and persistent pain relief and should be considered first-line surgical treatment for patients able to receive general anesthesia [47, 48]. Postoperative outcome was directly compared in 126 trigeminal neuralgia patients treated with a total of 153 separate surgical procedures: glycerol rhizotomy (N=51), stereotactic radiosurgery (N=69), or microvascular decompression (N=33) (Figure 4) [49]. Patients were followed for an average of two years after surgery. An excellent outcome was more likely to be achieved and maintained after microvascular decompression without additional treatment compared with the other two surgeries (P<0.01).

Table 18 Attributes of surgical treatments for trigeminal neuralgia.

	Short-term relief	Long-term relief	Complications
Rhizotomy	Good	Fair	Facial numbness and symptom recurrence
Stereotactic radiosurgery	Good	Good	Some facial paresthesia
Microvascular decompression	Excellent	Excellent	Minimal in addition to risks of general anesthesia

a. Immediate outcome

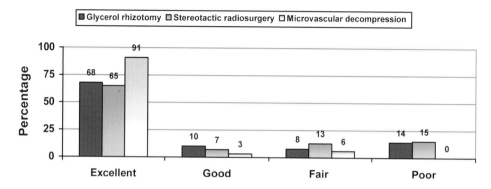

b. Long-term outcome

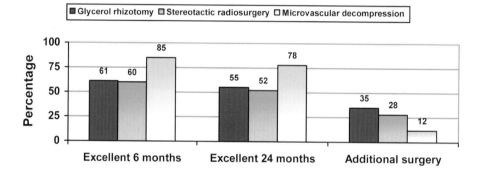

Figure 4 Surgical response with trigeminal neuralgia. a) Immediate outcome. b) Long-term outcome. An excellent response was assigned when patients reported no pain and usage of no medications. Good denoted no pain with low dose medication, fair >50% pain reduction and poor ≤50% pain reduction. (Based on Pollock 2005.)

Conclusions

Most patients for whom an uncommon headache diagnosis is considered will have an atypical presentation of a more common headache disorder rather than a rare headache. For this reason, all patients in whom an uncommon headache is being considered will need a full assessment to rule out more common diagnoses, including neuroimaging. In addition, new onset headache is not typically caused by a primary headache diagnosis in seniors. Although primary headaches that began in childhood or earlier adult years tend to improve with advancing age, one in five older adults report recurring headaches. Any new headache or change in headache pattern in older adults will require a detailed evaluation, including radiographic studies and often laboratory testing.

Key Summary

◆ Uncommon headaches affect <1% of the population.

◆ Basilar migraine and benign intracranial hypertension typically affect young females.

◆ Indomethacin-responsive headaches include hemicrania continua and paroxysmal hemicrania.

◆ SUNCT and SUNA are of very brief duration and are frequently recurring, unilateral headaches associated with autonomic symptoms.

◆ Giant cell arteritis is a medical emergency and early treatment is necessary to reduce the risk of permanent visual loss.

◆ Risk for post-herpetic neuralgia may be reduced by using zoster vaccination and early zoster treatment with antiviral or neuropathic medication.

◆ Trigeminal neuralgia failing to respond to medical therapy will be most effectively treated with microvascular decompression in patients able to tolerate general anesthesia.

References

1. Klapper J, Mathew N, Nett R. Triptans in the treatment of basilar migraine and migraine with prolonged aura. *Headache* 2001; 41: 981-984.
2. Asensio-Sánchez VM, Merino-Angulo J, Martínez-Calvo S, Calvo MJ, Rodríguez R. Epidemiology of pseudotumor cerebri. *Arch Soc Esp Oftalmol* 2007; 82: 219-221.
3. Galvin JA, Van Stavern GP. Clinical characterization of idiopathic intracranial hypertension at the Detroit Medical Center. *J Neurol Sci* 2004; 223: 157-160.
4. Rangwala LM, Liu GT. Pediatric idiopathic intracranial hypertension. *Surv Ophthalmol* 2007; 52: 597-617.
5. Camarda C, Camarda R, Monastero R. Chronic paroxysmal hemicrania and hemicrania continua responding to topiramate: two case reports. *Clin Neurol Neurosurg* 2008; 110: 88-91.
6. Lykke Thomsen L, Kirchmann Eriksen M, Faerch Romer S, *et al.* An epidemiological survey of hemiplegic migraine. *Cephalalgia* 2002; 22: 361-375.
7. Klapper J, Mathew N, Nett R. Triptans in the treatment of basilar migraine and migraine with prolonged aura. *Headache* 2001; 41: 981-984.
8. Artto V, Nissilä M, Wessman M, *et al.* Treatment of hemiplegic migraine with triptans. *Eur J Neurol* 2007; 14: 1053-1056.
9. Camarda C, Camarda R, Monastero R. Chronic paroxysmal hemicrania and hemicrania continua responding to topiramate: two case reports. *Clin Neurol Neurosurg* 2008; 110: 88-91.
10. Cohen AS, Matharu MS, Goadsby PJ. Short-lasting unilateral neuralgiform headache attacks with conjunctival injection and tearing (SUNCT) or cranial autonomic features (SUNA) - a prospective clinical study of SUNCT and SUNA. *Brain* 2006; 129: 2746-2760.
11. Cohen AS. Short-lasting unilateral neuralgiform headache attacks with conjunctival injection and tearing. *Cephalalgia* 2007; 27: 824-832.
12. Williams MH, Broadley SA. SUNCT and SUNA: clinical features and medical treatment. *J Clin Neurosci* 2008; 15: 526-534.
13. Camarda R, Monastero R. Prevalence of primary headaches in Italian elderly: preliminary data from the Zabút Aging Project. *Neurol Sci* 2003; 24: S122-S124.
14. Deleu D, Khan MA, Humaidan H, Al Mantheri Z, Al Hashami S. Prevalence and clinical characteristics of headache in medical students in Oman. *Headache* 2001; 41: 798-804.
15. González-Gay MA, Garcia-Porrua C, Rivas MJ, Rodriguez-Ledo P, Llorca J. Epidemiology of biopsy proven giant cell arteritis in northwestern Spain: trend over an 18-year period. *Ann Rheum Dis* 2001; 60: 367-371.
16. Salvarani C, Corwson CS, O'Fallon M, Hunder GG, Gabriel SE. Reappraisal of the epidemiology of giant cell arteritis in Olmsted County, Minnesota, over a fifty-year period. *Arthritis Rheum* 2004; 51: 264-268.
17. Salvarani C, Cantini F, Boiardi L, Hunder GG. Medical progress: polymyalgia rheumatica and temporal arteritis. *New Engl J Med* 2002; 347: 261-271.

18. Salvarini C, Cimino L, Macchioni P, *et al.* Risk factors for visual loss in an Italian population-based cohort of patients with giant cell arteritis. *Arthritis Care Res* 2005; 53: 293-297.

19. Gonzalez-Gay MA, Blanco R, Rodriguez-Valverde V, *et al.* Permanent visual loss and cerebrovascular accidents in giant cell arteritis. *Arthritis Rheum* 1998; 41: 1497-1504.

20. Pipitone N, Salvarani C. Improving therapeutic options for patients with giant cell arteritis. *Curr Opin Rheumatol* 2008; 20: 17-22.

21. Proven A, Gabriel SE, Orces C, O'Fallon M, Hunder GG. Glucocorticoid therapy in giant cell arteritis: duration and adverse outcomes. *Arthritis Care Res* 2003; 49: 703-708.

22. Evers S, Goadsby PJ. Hypnic headache. Clinical features, pathophysiology, and treatment. *Neurology* 2003; 60: 905-909.

23. Bowsher D. Postherpetic neuralgia and its treatment: a retrospective survey of 191 patients. *J Pain Symptom Manag* 1996; 12: 290-299.

24. Jung BF, Johnson RW, Griffin DR, Dworkin RH. Risk factors for postherpetic neuralgia in patients with herpes zoster. *Neurology* 2004; 62: 1545-1551.

25. Scott FT, Leedhan-Green ME, Barrett-Muir WY, *et al.* A study of shingles and the development of postherpetic neuralgia in East London. *J Med Virol* 2003; 70 (suppl 1): S24-S30.

26. Oxman MN, Levin MJ, Johnson GR, *et al.* A vaccine to prevent herpes zoster and postherpetic neuralgia in older adults. *N Engl J Med* 2005; 352: 2271-84.

27. Centers for Disease Control website: http://www.cdc.gov/vaccines/vpd-vac/shingles/default.htm. Accessed March 2008.

28. Gelb LD. Preventing herpes zoster through vaccination. *Ophthalmology* 2008; 115 (suppl): S35-S38.

29. Tyring S, Barbarash RA, Nahlik JE, *et al.* Famciclovir for the treatment of acute herpes zoster: effects on acute disease and postherpetic neuralgia. A randomized, double-blind, placebo-controlled trial. *Ann Intern Med* 1995; 123: 89-96.

30. Wassilew S. Brivudin compared with famciclovir in the treatment of herpes zoster: effects in acute disease and chronic pain in immunocompetent patients. A randomized, double-blind, multinational study. *J Eur Acad Dermatol Venereol* 2005; 19: 47-55.

31. Wassilew SW, Wutzler P. Oral brivudin in comparison with acyclovir for herpes zoster: a survey study on postherpetic neuralgia. *Antiviral Res* 2003; 59: 57-60.

32. Tyring SK, Beutner KR, Tucker BA, Anderson WC, Crooks RJ. Antiviral therapy for herpes zoster: randomized, controlled clinical trial of valacyclovir and famciclovir therapy in immunocompetent patients 50 years and older. *Arch Fam Med* 2000; 9: 863-869.

33. Bowsher D. The effects of pre-emptive treatment of postherpetic neuralgia with amitriptyline: a randomized, double-blind, placebo-controlled trial. *J Pain Symptom Manage* 1997; 13: 327-331.

34. Dubinsky RM, Kabbani H, El-Chami Z, *et al.* Practice parameter: treatment of postherpetic neuralgia: an evidence-based report of the Quality Standards Subcommittee of the American Academy of Neurology. *Neurology* 2004 ;63: 959-965.

35. Pappagallo M, Haldey EJ. Pharmacological management of postherpetic neuralgia. *CNS Drugs* 2003; 17: 771-780.

36. DeBeneditis G, Lorenzetti A. Topical aspirin/diethyl ether mixture versus indomethacin and diclofenac/diethyl ether mixture for acute herpetic neuralgia and postherpetic neuralgia: a double-blind, cross-over placebo controlled study. *Pain* 1996; 65: 45-51.

37. Katusic S, Beard CM, Bergstralh E, Kurland LT. Incidence and clinical features of trigeminal neuralgia, Rochester, Minnesota, 1945-1984. *Ann Neurol* 1990; 27: 89-95.

38. Hall GC, Carroll D, Parry D, McQuay HJ. Epidemiology and treatment of neuropathic pain: the UK primary care perspective. *Pain* 2006; 122: 156-162.

39. Chloe R, Patil R, Degwekar S, Bhowate R. Drug treatment of trigeminal neuralgia: a systematic review of the literature. *J Oral Maxillofac Surg* 2007; 65: 40-45.

40. Cheshire WP. Defining the role for gabapentin in the treatment of trigeminal neuralgia: a retrospective report. *J Pain* 2002; 3: 137-142.

41. Obermann M, Yoon MS, Sensen K, *et al*. Efficacy of pregabalin in the treatment of trigeminal neuralgia. *Cephalalgia* 2008; 28: 174-181.

42. Henson CF, Goldman HW, Rosenwasser RH, *et al*. Glycerol rhizotomy versus gamma knife radiosurgery for the treatment of trigeminal neuralgia: an analysis of patients treated at one institution. *Int J Radiat Oncol Biol Phys* 2005; 63: 82-90.

43. Jawahar A, Wadhwa R, Beck C, *et al*. Assessment of pain control, quality of life, and predictors of success after gamma knife surgery for the treatment of trigeminal neuralgia. *Neurosurg Focus* 2005; 18: E8.

44. Sheehan J, Pan HC, Stroila M, Steiner L. Gamma knife surgery for trigeminal neuralgia: outcomes and prognostic factors. *J Neurosurg* 2005; 102: 434-441.

45. Longhi M, Rizzo P, Nicolato A, *et al*. Gamma knife radiosurgery for trigeminal neuralgia: results and potentially predictive parameters - part I: idiopathic trigeminal neuralgia. *Neurosurgery* 2007; 61: 1254-1260.

46. Fountas KN, Smith JR, Lee GP, *et al*. Gamma knife stereotactic radiosurgical treatment of idiopathic trigeminal neuraliga: long-term outcome and complications. *Neurosurg Focus* 2007; 23: E8.

47. Sindou M, Leston J, Decullier E, Chapuis F. Microvascular decompression for primary trigeminal neuralgia: long-term effectiveness and prognostic factors in a series of 362 consecutive patients with clear-cut neurovascular conflicts who underwent pure decompression. *J Neurosurg* 2007; 107: 1144-1153.

48. Sindou M, Leston J, Howeidy T, Decullier E, Chapuis F. Micro-vascular decompression for primary trigeminal neuralgia (typical or atypical). Long-term effectiveness on pain; prospective study with survival analysis in a consecutive series of 362 patients. *Acta Neurochir (Wien)* 2006; 148:1235-1245.

49. Pollock BE, Ecker RD. A prospective cost-effectiveness study of trigeminal neuralgia surgery. *Clin J Pain* 2005; 21: 317-322.